BEYOND PAIN

CONQUER YOUR PAIN, RECLAIM YOUR LIFE

ANJELO RATNACHANDRA

Photocopying

Photocopying threatens the viability of future reprints. Vivid Publishing requests your compliance in ensuring the strategies contained in this unique resource are accessible by all through the approved points of sale.

Published by Vivid Publishing
A division of Fontaine Publishing Group
P.O. Box 948 Fremantle
Western Australia 6959
www.vividpublishing.com.au

National Library of Australia cataloguing-in-publication data:
Author: Ratnachandra, Anjelo, author.
Title: Beyond pain : conquer your pain, reclaim your life / Anjelo Ratnachandra.
ISBN: 9781925171693 (paperback)
Subjects: Pain--Treatment.
Dewey Number: 616.0472

Illustrations and diagrams: E. Alger, T. Hart
Cover design and text layout: Fontaine Publishing Group
Cover photographs: Zaleski Jayawardene and Meli James
Editor: Vikki Petraitis
Scientific Editor: Dr Gillian Dite

Disclaimer

All care has been taken in the preparation of the information herein. In view of ongoing research, the constant flow of information, changes in governmental regulations, differences in opinion amongst authorities, unique aspects of individual circumstances, and other factors, the reader is required to exercise judgement when making decisions regarding the information in this book, and compare and consult information from other sources. Neither the author nor the publisher may be held responsible or liable, howsoever, for any action, claim, issue, injury, loss or damage, resulting from the use of this book or any information contained within it. It is advised that the reader discuss the contents of this book with a specialist or health care practitioner before making use of this book.

The author would like to note that the vignettes used in this book comprises of mostly actual cases, some which are a collaboration of several cases, and some which are fictitious.

All contact details given in this book were current at the time of publication, but are subject to change.

www.beyondpain.com.au

'It's not what happens to you,
but how you react to it that matters.'
—Epictetus

This book is dedicated to people with chronic (persistent) pain. May you, within these pages, find the answers to all your questions, and the pathway to a better life.

ACKNOWLEDGEMENTS

Lying in a hospital bed with severe burns, it is hard to see the light at the end of the tunnel and hard to imagine that anything good could come from such a traumatic and painful event. Time not only healed my wounds, but it allowed me to learn from my experiences. I wouldn't wish what happened to me on my worst enemy, but that doesn't mean that I am not incredibly grateful for the things I have learnt from it. I am grateful that being a patient has made me a better clinician. I am grateful that I got the opportunity to view the world from a hospital bed.

As a physiotherapist, my greatest desire has always been to help people. Now, I hope that by sharing my story and my understandings, people in pain can use these methods to reduce their pain and live better lives.

While I have spent years working one-to-one with people, the book version of my Beyond Pain program was untested until volunteers started coming in droves, offering to trial it. It has now become an award winning program.

I would like to thank those people for their invaluable feedback, which helped shape and refine the program into the success it is today. It is gratifying to see the Beyond Pain program stand on its own, and help so many people to overcome their pain.

It's hard to know exactly what to thank your parents for when they have given you so much: values, education, support, encouragement, curries, ironing, advice and love. To Ranjith and Ramya, the best parents a man could have, thank you for everything.

To my siblings, thank you for your daily phone calls and for helping Mum and Dad to visit me in London.

When you're overseas and can't have your family by your side, relatives can be the next best thing. For taking me into their hearts and their home, and for treating me like a son and brother, I would like to thank my Uncle Jine, Aunty Mal, Saj and Nadie.

A friend in need is a friend indeed. When I was in need, suffering severe burns, unable to do much for myself, my friends came to my side without a moment's hesitation. My sincere thanks go to Chan, Anita, Jill, Duncan, and all my other friends and relatives who braved London's weather and transport system to visit me regularly, bringing food and good cheer. I am indebted to you.

Thanks also to my colleagues from Input Pain Management who supported me through my rehabilitation process, especially my manager, Vicky Harding.

Thank you to Nola Chapman, whose encouragement drove me to write this book.

To the following friends and colleagues: Prof Francis J Keefe, Dr Toby Newton-John, Dr Jacqui Stanford, Dr Prue Lewis, Emily Woods, Melinda Hickey, Luke Hickey, Amanda Ide, Holly Foura, Vanessa Edwards, Thilina De Silva, Trish Edwards, Kristie-Lee King, Brendan McCormack, Sammani Dharmatilleka, Lauren McCormack, Lizzy Walton, Carina Enea, and Ella Collins, thank you for your support during the development of these pages.

I would like to thank author Vikki Petraitis who mentored me through the uncharted waters of writing a book. You helped to make my vision of sharing my knowledge a reality.

And last, but certainly not least, I'd like to thank my wife, Vin. Your unwavering encouragement, support and energy were instrumental in my recovery and in the writing of this book. Without you, I would be a very different man in a very different place.

ABOUT THE AUTHOR

Anjelo Ratnachandra was born in Sri Lanka and immigrated to Australia as a child to escape a brutal civil war. Ratnachandra and his family made their home in Glen Waverley, what was then a quiet suburb of Melbourne. He excelled in high school and later graduated from the University of Melbourne with honours before beginning his career as a Physiotherapist. Ratnachandra broadened his knowledge and experience in Physiotherapy by working in private and public clinics in Australia and overseas.

While overseas he pursued his interest in pain management, and after returning to Australia in 2007, he began working in Occupational Rehabilitation. In 2008, he founded Beyond Pain, one of the first private practice chronic pain physiotherapy services in Australia. Beyond Pain has since grown to be more than just a chronic pain service; it also helps people with chronic fatigue and mental illnesses.

Ratnachandra is one of only a few practitioners in the world holding a dual qualification in Physiotherapy and Counselling. He is an award-winning practitioner who has been recognised for his clinical and occupational rehabilitation work. He has assisted in pain studies run by the University of Melbourne and Deakin University (Melbourne), and, has developed ground-breaking concepts such as the *Pain Street-Map Analogy*, the *Life Triad*, and the *Hierarchy of Being*. Further, he has pioneered tel-ehealth, helping clients all over Australia and overseas through videoconferencing. Aside from his clinical and coaching work, Ratnachandra also works with organisations developing wellbeing programs, and, is a popular keynote speaker.

Today, Ratnachandra lives with his family in regional Victoria. He continues to be well respected by his peers and recognised for his work. His vision is to share his knowledge, in particular, his successful pain management program with sufferers all over the world; a vision he is determined to make a reality.

CONTENTS

Part 1 – The Journey

Part 2 – The Understanding

Part 3 – Beyond Pain Program

PART 1
THE JOURNEY

INTRODUCTION

Over the many years working in pain management, I have come to learn that pain can manifest in many forms. It may be sharp, dull or an annoying ache. It may feel like electric shocks, or like broken glass under your skin. It may have been there for a few weeks or for several decades.

I have also learnt that the events that cause pain can vary too. It may be something as simple as bending over to pick up a pen, or just playing ball with your kids. It may be a gradual build up with no incident at all. For me, it was a sudden and horrific event, but for you, this may not be the case.

Not that it matters, because the result is exactly the same.

Pain.

Pain affects us all differently. While some have achieved amazing feats despite their pain, you may be just trying to make it through each day. Things most people take for granted, like getting up out of bed, taking a shower, or just trying to watch a favourite TV show, might be agonising for you.

But irrespective of the kind of pain you have, how bad it is or how you got it, pain is pain. It is not something you want, but something you have to deal with.

And whether your pain is worse than mine, or not so bad, it doesn't matter – we both have pain. Some people have found it hard to relate to my story because of the extraordinary events that led to my pain. Nevertheless, I found a way to conquer my pain and achieve my goals, using strategies that anyone can use.

This is my story. It's about not giving up; it's about knowing that if you want something badly enough, there is a way. By reading this book, you will be able to learn from my knowledge and experiences, and succeed in achieving your goals, using the simple strategies that have worked for me.

This book may just contain the answers you're looking for.

MY BIG ADVENTURE

I caught the travel bug. That's how I, Anjelo Ratnachandra, a Melbourne-raised Sri Lankan immigrant came to be working in the heart of London. I landed in London five days shy of my twenty-fifth birthday. And, to the joy of my ridiculously proud parents, I was working as a qualified physiotherapist.

But if the truth be told, the travel bug had bitten years earlier. In Year 11, I was chosen to be an exchange student for three weeks in China. Other than that and two trips to visit family in Sri Lanka, the furthest I'd been from my home had been holidays in Apollo Bay with my aunty and uncle. Most other holidays, I worked to help my parents with the mortgage on our humble suburban home in Glen Waverley.

In the Ratnachandra family, education is important. Mum and Dad gave up an affluent lifestyle in Sri Lanka to give us the opportunities that Australia had to offer. At the time, the brutal civil war became too much for them. Schools were often closed because of bomb threats and that limited our opportunities. Mum and Dad left a nice home and highly paid positions in marketing, not to mention the three maids and the chauffeur, to bring my older brother, Arjuna, my younger sister, Ranmali, and me to Melbourne. You only have to spend five minutes with my parents to know that their children come first.

My parents' sacrifice came with a cost. In Australia, their lack of formal qualifications meant factory jobs and a hardship they hadn't known before. There were even days when we took buttered bread for school lunch because pay-day hadn't arrived yet. Despite this, their grace and humility, coupled with their desire to give their children a better life in a world without bombs, meant that we never once heard them complain. We assimilated into Australian life without many gaffes, except for the time when Mum sent me to a casual clothes day at primary school dressed as an army soldier.

To repay our parents, Arjuna, Ranmali and I worked as hard as we could at school. I was dux a number of times and finished Year 12 with a score of 98.45 out of a possible 99.95. The day I was accepted to Melbourne University, Mum and Dad rang family and friends in Sri Lanka so that they could boast long distance. If there were prouder parents anywhere in the world, it would have been surprising. My parents weren't proud of my score, they were proud of me. They had seen me labouring through holiday jobs – doing paper rounds and even helping the janitor at my school – any job that I could get my hands on, just to help buy my books.

I put the same effort into tertiary study that I had at school. At twenty-two, I graduated with honours as a physiotherapist. What I loved about the practical side of my work was that I could see people, treat them and see them walk away better off after my intervention.

During my training, I saw physiotherapists pushed for time and over-worked. Worse than that, there were patients not getting the service that they should have. I also saw long waiting lists at public hospitals for patients in pain. Over the four years of my course, I decided that when I finished, I wanted to open my own business and provide a prompt service to a high standard.

With my graduation certificate in one hand and the key to my clinic – a single room in a busy Noble Park medical centre – in the other, I opened my own business and slowly built up my clientele while supporting myself by working in other clinics as well. While I felt that I could help most people, there were repeat customers who gained no more than temporary relief from my treatments. They'd walk out telling me they felt better, but a couple of days later they'd be back. It was these sufferers of chronic pain that presented the greatest challenges for me. I did everything I knew how to do, but long-term, I didn't feel I could offer them much.

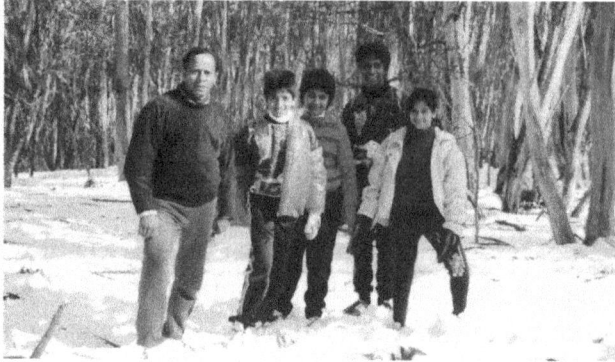

Our first family trip to the snow

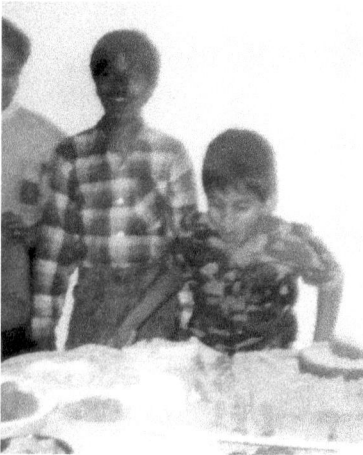

My 10th birthday

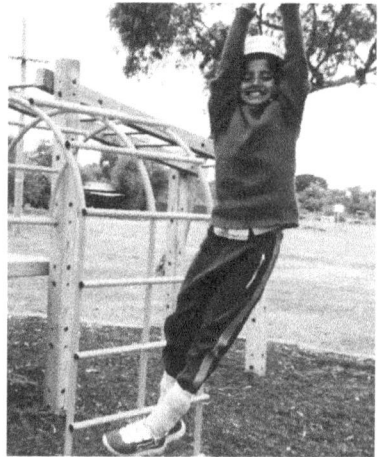

Me having fun in the park

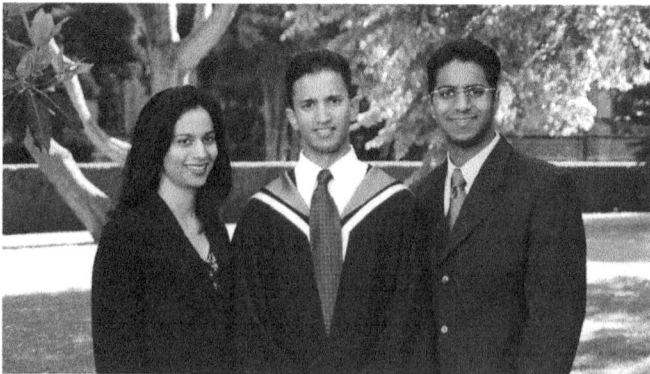

Graduation day with Ranmali (left) and Arjuna (right)

While I felt a bit helpless, these patients intrigued me. Everyone put them in the too-hard basket. I didn't want to do that, but I wasn't sure what I had to do. I knew that whatever treatment they needed must include a psychological component as well. I would often hear statements like: 'my grandkids came over the other day and we had such a great time playing that I forgot about my pain' or 'I went out for the day with my friends and we walked around a flower show. I didn't even notice my bad back.' The psychological component simply couldn't be overlooked.

Fermenting in my understanding was the idea that their treatment did not begin and end in my twenty-minute sessions with them. There was a clear link between mood and having a purpose. Self-belief made a big difference too. But in those early days when I was working 70-hour weeks, I had little time to follow these seeds of understanding with any formal study. For now, it was all anecdotal, but there were definite patterns in patients, particularly those with chronic pain.

After a year or so of having a social life comparable to a monk, I made a decision that would change everything. I closed the doors of my clinic, quit my other physio jobs, and booked a ticket to London. I decided that because London was the centre of everywhere, I could see the world a bit at a time, and eventually arrive at my ultimate destination: Mt Everest base camp. I had always imagined the Himalayas to be the pinnacle, the top of the world. And most importantly to me, the Himalayas represented a destination where my faith, Buddhism, was at home among the soaring mountains, isolated towns and yak-worn paths winding through rocky outcrops.

I could finance my travels by working as a physio in London. A few of my friends from university had done it, and hearing them talk about places like Prague, Paris and Rome being close enough for a weekend trip had awoken my dormant travel bug.

Mum was worried by my decision. None of her children had spent much time away from home. Dad wasn't much better; they were both a pair of worry-warts. Mum was sure someone would attack me on the streets of London and that I would lie unconscious in a gutter, and then how could she ever forgive herself for letting me go? Dad didn't reveal his own doomsday scenarios about me and gutters, but he nodded vigorously whenever Mum recited hers. His silence and worried frowns spoke volumes.

The fact that Mum actually let go of me at the airport was a minor miracle. She was clutching her tissues and me in equal measures. After Mum's crying, I was kind of relieved to get on the plane. I was just short of turning twenty-five, but I might as well have been twelve as far as Mum was concerned.

London never sleeps. A million miles away from my Glen Waverley upbringing, I was like a kid in a candy shop, taking everything in. It was surreal to see the places I had only ever seen in pictures: Parliament House, Big Ben, Buckingham Palace and Tower Bridge.

At Mum's insistence, I moved in with my Dad's second cousin's family in Orpington, Kent. Aunty Mal, Uncle Jine, their son Saj and daughter Nadie were great, but before long, it was a bit like being at home with Mum and Dad, and I craved independence. Before I left Australia, I had organised a job through an agency. I was a community physiotherapist, driving around in a work car to visit patients. Most were elderly people who had suffered a stroke or had recently had surgery. It was a great way of seeing Kent, which is known as the garden of England. One of my patients had a garden that had been voted one of the best in Kent. It had little bridges over a stream with hills in the background, and a riot of flowers lined a winding driveway, backed by perfectly trimmed hedges. It was like something from a movie.

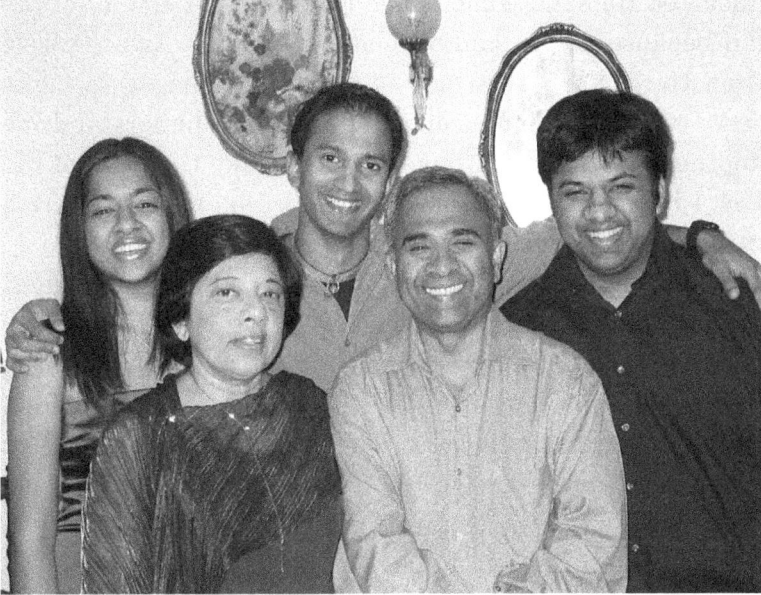

My UK family from left, Nadie, aunty Mal, uncle Jine, and Saj

When my contract ended, I wanted to expand my horizons from relatives and lush gardens to the vibrant life in London. My university buddies had spoken fondly of their share-house experiences and I started to look for something closer to the city. Uncle Jine's house was like living in Melbourne's quiet leafy Camberwell when you've wanted to live in cosmopolitan St Kilda.

My first share-house wasn't so much a house but a tiny two-bedroom flat on a council estate that might have been featured on *The Bill*. Probably was for all I know. There were seven of us. I was the only one fluent in English,

sharing a very cramped space with three Chinese people,
a Korean guy and a Russian couple. I felt like the United
Nations – always being called in to settle arguments between
the volatile housemates. Everyone cooked for themselves
and access to the kitchen had to be scheduled into time
slots. There was always a curry that took longer than the
allocated time. Or some boiled cabbage that smelt out the
flat because no one had opened the window. As an Aussie
from the suburbs, I'm not sure how I managed to make
sense of what was going on and make them understand one
another. By the end of my stay, I felt like the head of the
UN. I lasted twelve months before fleeing to somewhere a
little bigger than a closet to call home.

It was around this time in July 2005 that I got a job at
a program operating at St Thomas' Hospital called Input
Pain Management. Physiotherapy in its pure form is very
hands on – patients come, we massage, we manipulate,
we set exercises and try our best to fix their ailments. But
every day, there were people for whom this didn't work.
That was why the Input Pain Management program
made such an impact on me. The program wasn't about a
hands-on approach. It offered people advice and strategies
to cope with long-term pain. I got a job at the program,
keen to fill the deficit in my professional knowledge.

The training dictated that we script our group treatment
sessions. It gave me support while I learned a new way of
helping people, and I valued the safety-net. But I sometimes
found myself referring to things I didn't understand. One
exercise was a stretch that we had to say was 'like a Kenny
Everett'. I had no idea who or what a Kenny Everett
was. Someone later told me that he was a comedian. The
exercise was a leg-crossing while lying down that looked
more like Sharon Stone to me. But we couldn't deviate
from the script so it stayed a Kenny Everett.

By day, I helped people and made Kenny Everett references that I didn't understand, and by night I expanded my growing social circles. Uni buddies from Australia, work buddies, friends I met through other friends, and one Sri Lankan guy I really clicked with whom I met at the Buddhist temple in Kent. His name was Chan. He was a couple of years older than me and had a dry, witty sense of humour. We went to parties and clubs, and sometimes even tried to chat up girls, but neither of us was very good at it. He was my wingman, but he kept insisting that I was his.

My second share-house experience in a house full of smokers didn't work out when I woke up one morning with a pain in my chest.

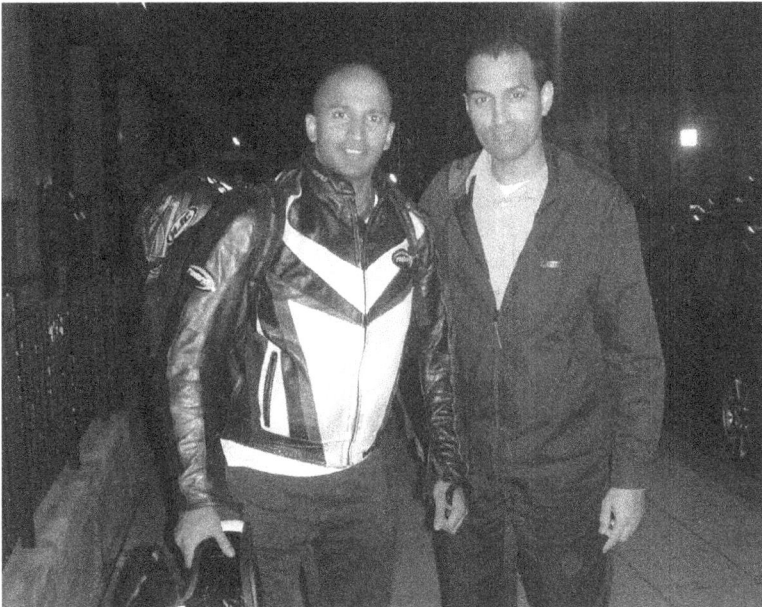

Hitting the bars in London

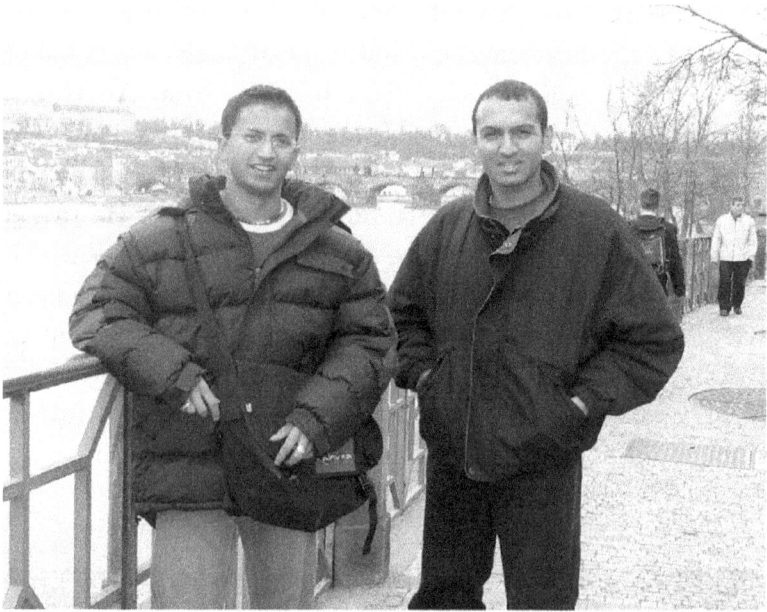

My trip to Prague

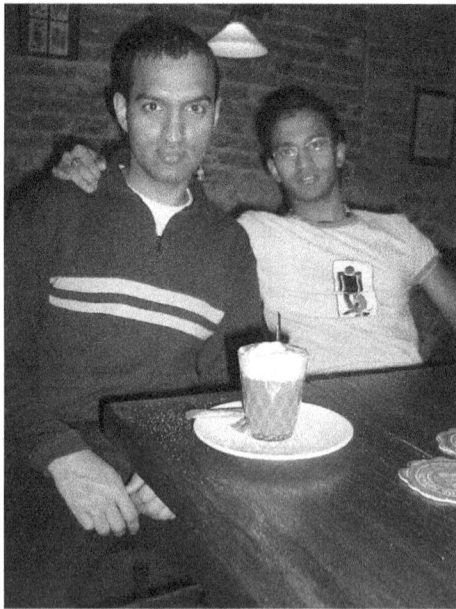

A lazy Sunday arvo catch up with Chan

THE FIRST BLIP ON THE RADAR

I have never smoked, and neither has anyone in my family. At first, living in a house full of smokers made me cough, but like anything in life, you get used to stuff over time. And pretty soon, I hardly noticed the smell of cigarette smoke that clung to every stick of furniture and every thread of clothing that I owned. Aside from the phlegmy cough that I suffered each morning when I woke up in my pungent environment, I figured that because I wasn't home much anyway, it was hardly likely that I would suffer from long-term passive smoking symptoms.

On Tuesday 25 October 2005, I was at rugby training as the team physio. I loved watching the game from the sidelines and looked forward to hanging out at the clubhouse bar to down a few beers.

Towards the end of the training session, the ball flew out of bounds right towards me, and as I reached to catch it, I felt a pull in my ribs and flinched. For a moment, it was like a stitch and I figured that I had strained one of my intercostals – the muscles between my ribs. No big deal.

Later that night, I met up with a mate. He noticed that I kept rubbing my side and asked what had happened. I laughed as I told him that I had probably just pulled a muscle and I hadn't even been playing. I noticed that I was a bit short of breath as I told him my short story of injury.

My mate, who played rugby for another team, said that

I might have a collapsed lung.

'Don't be so melodramatic,' I laughed.

My alarm went off the next morning, and as I reached for it, a pain shot through me that felt like someone had stabbed me in the chest. I managed to turn off the alarm and sat up. My breathing quickened into a childbirth type pant. I clutched my side. The muscle I'd pulled the night before was seriously hurting me. I struggled to the kitchen and grabbed some Panadol. It took me almost an hour to get showered and dressed – triple the time it normally took.

On the train to work, I knew the Panadol wasn't even touching the pain. I figured that I would have to just ride it out. I don't like taking too many painkillers and normally avoid them altogether if I can.

From the Westminster tube station, it was a short walk across the bridge to St Thomas' Hospital where I worked. The walk, which normally took five minutes, took me nearly half an hour because I had to keep stopping to catch my breath. It was like my lungs couldn't get enough air. And every time I took a deep breath, I had a sharp pain in my side.

When I finally got to work, I told one of my Aussie nurse friends that I had a pain in the side of my chest.

'Stop whinging Anj,' she said. 'You're sounding like a girl.' With a pat on my back, she walked off grinning.

I struggled through the whole day. One of our occupational therapists, who had a disability that made her hobble, came over and checked on me at the end of the day.

'Are you all right, Anj?' she asked concerned. 'You're walking slower than me.'

I told her about my strained side and that I was having difficulty breathing.

'Maybe you should get one of the doctors here to check you out.'

Normally, I would have avoided that, but there was something about the way I was feeling... maybe it would be best for a doctor to examine me and reassure me that it was just a strained muscle.

It was early evening by the time I got to see the doctor. She listened to my chest, tapped my side and told me that it was probably not a collapsed lung because I didn't fit the criteria. Tall thin teenagers are usually the main sufferers of this because their skeletons grow quicker than their internal tissue, causing tension. While I was thin, I wasn't tall and I wasn't a teenager.

The doctor said that if it didn't improve in a couple of days, I should go for an X-ray.

Over the next couple of days, I came into work. I got used to being slightly out of breath and convinced myself that I would be fine. I had planned a trip to Budapest with some friends for the next weekend and I really wanted to feel better by then.

Our flight was scheduled for late Friday afternoon and I carried a backpack to work with me. I was in agony by the time I got there, but being a bloke bound for Budapest, I ignored each and every one of my symptoms.

When the seatbelt sign came on as the plane took off, the pain was so severe that I had to leave my seat and crawl into the aisle and stretch out my arm to try and get relief in my chest and neck. From his seated position in the stewards' section, one of the male flight attendants looked at me with horror, his eyes like saucers. With equal horror, I realised what I must look like. It was just after the London bombings, and here I was acting weird on my knees, out in the aisle when the seat belt signs were on. I quickly climbed back into my seat and reassured him.

'I'm only stretching, mate,' I said. 'Sorry!'

He looked marginally relieved and sort of smiled at me.

Sitting for an hour in a pressurised cabin puts a lot of pressure on your chest. If your chest is healthy, you don't normally notice the pressure. When there's something wrong, you notice it: a lot.

By the time we landed, the friends I was travelling with – some of whom were health professionals themselves – all concluded that I had a collapsed lung.

'Nah, it can't be,' I told them with more conviction than I felt. 'Let's just enjoy the weekend. I'll be fine.'

I put the day's pain down to the fact that I hadn't carried a backpack for a while and that I must have aggravated my sore muscle. Talk about denial.

Budapest was a beautiful historic city. My friends and I walked the cobbled streets, ate at little cafes and enjoyed the brightly-coloured markets. It was a place to walk around, rather than drive. Our group walked at a comfortable pace, enjoying the scenery.

'I think I'm getting better,' I told the group after walking around most of Saturday with not a lot of discomfort.

'No, you're not!' said one of my mates. 'You're still panting like a steam train and walking like an old man.'

I was so busy ignoring my symptoms that I hadn't thought for a moment that they were completely obvious to my mates.

That night, we all hit the local disco. It was like stepping back into 1975 – mirror balls and weird music – but it was the only place we could find. Packed in like sardines, we all had a couple of drinks. I had my usual Scotch and Coke but it hit me like a mallet. After two drinks, my head was spinning along with the mirror ball, and I switched to straight Coke.

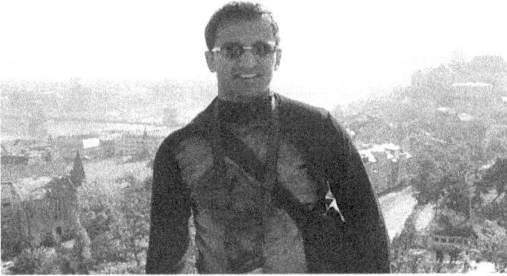

A disaster waiting to happen

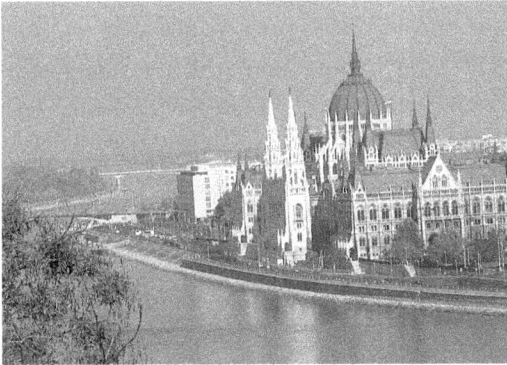

Beautiful Budapest

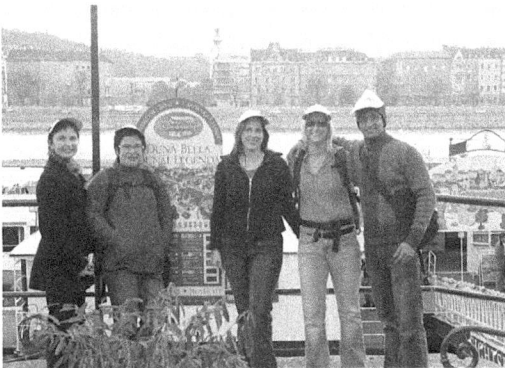

My travel mates from left, Julie, Polly, Kate, and Lesley

On the return flight home, I didn't feel as bad and assumed I was on the road to recovery. I was exhausted and had a very early night.

The next morning, I woke up and realised that the pain in my side was gone. I took a deep breath and nearly choked. I coughed a phlegmy cough and started to worry. I was still short of breath and now this cough, when I haven't got a cold, made me nervous. Professionally, if I had a patient with these symptoms, I would suspect pneumonia.

I rang work to tell them I'd be late, and then went to my own local doctor. After tapping and listening to my chest, the doctor suggested that I might have tuberculosis, which was common among the immigrant population where I was living.

'Doc, I don't have TB. I'm Australian,' I told him. 'I'm a physio. Can you give me an X-ray slip and I'll go get it checked out.'

Armed with my X-ray referral, I caught the train down to the local hospital. The guy who did the X-ray then sent me to wait in the waiting room for the results. Five minutes later, he ran out.

'Do you need an ambulance?' he asked urgently.

'Um…' Confusion. 'Why?'

'You have a large pneumo-thorax. You need to get to emergency right now!' He ushered me into a cubicle and showed me my X-rays on the light box.

My right lung was normal, but my left lung looked like a deflated balloon, all weird and pear-shaped.

'Don't worry about the ambulance,' I told him, figuring that it would be quicker to walk up the road to the Royal London than to wait for an ambulance to battle the traffic. I took my X-rays in an envelope and set off up the road.

I expected that the treatment would involve the doctor inserting a syringe and removing the excess air in the cavity so that my lung could inflate again. Simple, I thought.

I was wrong.

I admitted myself into Accident and Emergency, and before long, I was surrounded by a group of medical students and their supervising doctor.

'So you have no history of this? Nothing in the family?' asked the doctor.

'No,' I replied.

'It says here you flew twice within seventy-two hours?' he asked sternly.

'Um, I guess so.' I felt like a child waiting to be told off.

'Do you realise that the worst thing you could do with a collapsed lung is deep-sea dive or fly?' He gave me a very disapproving look.

'Well at least I didn't deep-sea dive as well,' I said lamely.

'Looking at the X-rays, your left lung has collapsed to less than 40%. You probably had about forty-eight hours before collapsing dead on the street.'

What? Thank God I didn't deep-sea dive.

'We will need to use a syringe to take the air out of the cavity so it's not pressing on your lung. Are you happy for one of the students to do it?'

'Er... I guess I don't mind.' I appreciated that students have to learn, because that's how I learnt. But when you're on the wrong end of a very long needle, and you could have been dead on a street within forty-eight hours, I really hoped he picked an A-grade student to wield the needle.

The student turned out to be a confident young woman, but despite removing a litre of air from my chest cavity, my left lung refused to inflate and reseal the cavity. The doctor took over and inserted a chest catheter and told me that all should be right in a couple of days.

'We see this all the time,' he said without any concern.

A week passed and a steady stream of friends and relatives visited me in hospital. As each day passed, my concerns grew. The doctors didn't seem to be too worried, but I wasn't sure if they had a good grasp of the situation. They kept saying that a collapsed lung should fix itself in a couple of days, but a week on, there was no improvement. Maybe I needed to be in a specialist ward.

Finally, one of the doctors explained that they were going to transfer me to the London Chest Hospital.

'Why?' I asked with equal measures of relief and concern: relief that I was going to a specialist hospital and concern because I needed to.

'We don't really know why your lung hasn't fully inflated. We just want you to be under specialist care, so it would be the best option to go there,' he said.

At the London Chest Hospital, they took out the small catheter and replaced it with a much larger one. After a week, things looked much brighter and the doctors were confident that my lung had fully inflated. They removed the tube and I felt relieved.

I was packing my bags to go home when a young doctor arrived and told me that they had decided to keep me in for one more night to monitor my progress. Hospitals are like a black hole – just when you think you can leave, you are sucked back into their vacuum. With an impatient sigh, I undressed, put my PJs back on and climbed back into bed. An impatient patient.

Nonetheless, my mood picked up. I even got my appetite back and willingly ate a dinner of soggy fish and chips from the hospital kitchen. That night, as I closed my eyes, I smiled to myself. This would be the most comfortable night that I had experienced since my lung collapsed. Now that the tube was removed, I could roll over as I pleased, free as a bird. I drifted off.

Waking disoriented in the darkened ward, I squinted to try to read the time on my watch. It was 3.30 in the morning. And I was in pain. I took in a deep breath and *pop*. My heart was racing and I felt like I was being choked.

Oh no, my lung had collapsed again. I could feel it. *No.* A storm of emotions went through me: disappointment, anger, helplessness and disbelief. I pressed the call buzzer. The nurse came to my bedside and agreed with my self-diagnosis. She immediately organised a mobile X-ray machine that also agreed with my diagnosis. My left lung was like a punctured balloon.

Later that morning, when a doctor explained that I needed surgery, I only had one question for him.

'Doc, do you think I can still trek the Himalayas?'

'If everything goes smoothly and you stay fit and active, you could...' she paused. 'But you have to understand, there is always a risk of it collapsing again. There is less oxygen at those altitudes. Your lungs will have to work a lot harder. If you're fit enough and you pace yourself, there's no reason you couldn't. Of course, after surgery, you do realise that you won't even be allowed on a plane for three months, don't you? So you won't be doing anything any time soon.'

All I wanted was a chance, and she gave that to me.

After saying that I needed surgery, the doctor told me that I would be put on a waiting list. In the meantime, a new catheter was inserted to inflate my lung. Again.

It took another week. A steady stream of friends and relatives continued to make a beeline for my bedside. Luckily, they brought food along with their company. Three weeks of soggy London hospital food was making me gag; after that long, it all looks and smells the same. My aunt and uncle from Kent, Uncle Jine and Aunty Mal, brought in some home-cooked Sri Lankan food, which smelt like heaven and tasted just as good. They are both in the medical profession – he is an anaesthetist and she is a psychiatrist. My best mate Chan's mum would travel an hour on public transport to bring me a selection of fruit and home-cooked Sri Lankan food. I couldn't believe how fortunate I was to have such amazing friends and relatives. Together, we laughed and joked. My workmates entertained me with visits and I would chide them.

'So much for your diagnostic skills, you told me to stop whinging,' I said, pointing to my chest tube.

'See, still whinging,' they would say, handing me the chocolate milkshake I had asked them to get me on the way in.

After three weeks of lying around, eating brought-in food and laughing with my mates, when the doctor finally appeared by my bedside to explain the surgery I was going to have, I was ill-prepared for his last question.

'Have you made a Will?' he asked.

A what? A Will? Might I die?

'No...' I said.

He left my bedside after advising me that now would be a good time to make one.

My world narrowed from the ward and zoomed into just me. For a moment, it was like I was alone floating in the universe. I closed my eyes and sat in my self-imposed darkness. Is this my last day on earth? If it was, did I have regrets? Could I have fitted anything else in? I thought of loving my family, studying, working hard to get where I was, travelling, seeing the world, the freedom of riding my motorbike in and around London, and finally, I thought about the work that I was doing to help people in pain.

No. I didn't regret a thing.

I had packed as much into my life as I possibly could. I

would regret not having a future, if I did die, but I wouldn't regret the past. The only pang I suffered was not reaching the Himalayas.

And then my conscious mind took over. My eyes opened to the light. All surgery carried a risk – I knew that – but the risk was low. I needed to be practical about it. I reached for the notebook I kept next to my bed and thought about what I owned and who I would leave it to. Luckily, my list was fairly short: a five-year-old motorbike, a very old car, clothes and a hardly-used guitar that I'd been meaning to learn to play. I also owned a small portion – probably the driveway – of an investment property back home in Wantirna; Mum and Dad would get that. Chan could have the old car back because he had given it to me in the first place. It only took a couple of minutes and one sheet of my notepad to divvy up my meagre belongings to friends and family. It occurred to me that a life lived to the full doesn't amount to much on paper.

On paper, I was worth very little, but I knew that my purpose-filled life, lived to overflowing, was worth millions. And I was worth a lot to the stream of family and friends who, daily, visited with food and laughter and love.

Having surgery is like being kidnapped by aliens. On those dodgy documentaries that we have all watched, there is always a bloke from the Deep South in America describing how he saw a bright light, and then experienced 'lost time' and figured that he had been taken to the mothership and probed. Surgery is like that. One minute you are awake, the next minute your eyes are flickering open and you have no sense of time passing at all. And it's all over. And you're not dead.

After my lost time, I awoke to the sound of monitors beeping and the *psshhh* sound of oxygen flowing through the mask strapped to my face. I knew I was still alive because of the pain. I fell back asleep surrounded by tubes and machines.

Later, I woke up feeling slightly more alert; Uncle Jine and Aunty Mal had arrived with my cousin Nadie.

'So, what should I tell your parents?' my uncle asked, frowning.

'Tell them that everything was fine,' I replied instinctively. I had tried to protect my parents from what was going on. *Oh it's only a collapsed lung*, I had told them when all this started. *Happens to lots of people. It's nothing. No, of course you don't have to fly all the way over here. I'll be fine. It's just a small operation. Nothing really. I'll be back on my feet in no time.*

So I had lied to them. My beloved parental worry-warts would have been on the first plane to London had they any idea of how serious my condition was. And that wouldn't have been a good thing. I had to put all my energy into getting well. I didn't have any to spare to keep them calm and stop them from kidnapping me from the hospital, carrying me to the roof of the hospital to a waiting helicopter piloted by a friend of Dad's cousin's next-door neighbour to take me to a waiting charter plane that they had mortgaged their house to hire to fly me back to the safety of Melbourne. Or something like that.

But my uncle was more honest than me.

'I'm not going to lie to them,' said Uncle Jine. Being a doctor, he no doubt had realised the seriousness of my condition, even though I had kept it from him too.

The fight went out of me. 'Fine. Tell them what you think they need to know... depending on how they're reacting.'

Uncle Jine knew what Mum and Dad were like; they knew what all Sri Lankan parents were like – crazy and whacky where their children were concerned. He'd be hiring a helicopter for a roof kidnapping if this was his daughter Nadie or his son Sajith. He nodded.

It took Mum and Dad a week from hearing the news to be standing by my bed. Weeping. Well, Mum was weeping, Dad was stroking my hand.

'What did we do to make this happen to you?' wailed Mum.

'Mum, you did nothi–'

'We've always tried to be good parents,' wept Mum.

'Mum, I'm ok–'

'Don't worry. We're here now. We can take care of you,' said Dad, looking at all my tubes and machines as if he should make an adjustment.

'Dad, it's all righ–'

'Don't worry, Son, we're not going to leave your sight until you're fully recovered.'

Oh God...

The tears I cried when they finally left the hospital at the end of the day were partly the build-up of frustration from being in hospital for four weeks, and partly because I'd flown around the world to gain independence and now I felt like I was ten years old again.

When the machines were finally disconnected from me (although the tubes were still in), I knew it was important to do any exercise that I could to build up the fitness that I had lost. I had to practice the same principles that I preached to my patients. Exercise would also give my lungs a workout and help with the healing process. Soon after the surgery, I was able to spend ten minutes on an exercise bike and I did this five times a day. I tried to walk up and down near my bed and jog on the spot.

My journey to the Himalayas depended on getting fit. That kept me motivated.

By the end of the first week after surgery – a month in hospital – I woke up one day and didn't feel like any more visitors. I just wanted to be left alone. Being happy and smiling was now an effort. I'd rather stay alone and drown myself in my own thoughts. *Why is this happening to me? Am I ever going to get out of here? And will they ever remove these bloody tubes from my chest?* Surprisingly, self-pity came quite naturally. Upbeat, joking Anj was now wallowing in self-pity.

You can't stop family and friends from visiting, and of course, Mum and Dad's daily bedside vigil was mandatory. While I tried to put on a happy face, frustration began leaking into their visits. I would snap at them, and at the nurses, as if I couldn't help myself. But mostly, my visitors sensed something was wrong because of my silence. I had run out of things to say. For now, I was just waiting. Waiting for seven words.

'We are taking out your tubes today,' said a doctor, one fine day.

Ahhh, the very seven words I'd been waiting to hear. Sweet.

On 4 December 2005, I packed my bags, thanked the staff for looking after me and hurried outside to get away before they had any chance of telling me that I couldn't go. After almost five weeks of the unchanging hospital temperature, the chill of the winter breeze was like a tonic as I stepped out the electronic doors to freedom. Christmas decorations in the streets added to the feeling of festivity.

I spent the next month living at my uncle and aunt's place along with Mum and Dad. Luckily, I was able to go back to work pretty much straight away, so while I was fussed over and cooked for at night, during the day I could feel like a normal, functioning, working, busy member of society. I was so happy that I could almost ignore coming home to crisply folded undies, perfectly matched socks, delicious home-cooked meals and five thousand questions about my health and whether their parenting had anything to do with my lung collapse.

I knew I couldn't go back to my old place. I gave notice to the smokers that I would be moving out and then set about finding a smoke-free house to share.

Celebrating a white Christmas at my uncle's house in Kent was a turkey and plum-pudding-filled conclusion to the event of my collapsed lung. The doctors didn't know what caused it, whether or not it could happen again, or whether my life could return to normal. Apart from the three-month embargo on flying or deep-sea diving, I could pretty much do whatever I wanted. And what I really wanted to do was to show my parents I was well, wave goodbye to them at the airport, find a new place to live and get on with my life.

THIRD TIME'S A CHARM

Third time lucky. I ended up in a great house in Bow with two Aussies, Anita and Jill, and a girl from upstate New York called Lauren. They were the perfect housemates – kind, generous, thoughtful, normal, and importantly, non-smokers. Anita, although she was younger than me, took on the mothering role in the house. She kept an eye on bills and budgets, and made sure everyone pulled their weight. She was a teacher, and organising us all came naturally. Jill was the youngest by a few years, a free spirit who made decisions on a whim. Lauren was a soft-hearted soul who laughed at our dry Aussie sense of humour and sarcasm even if she didn't get a lot of our quips, just so she didn't offend us. The only time she fired up was when any of us opposed her views – then we saw evidence of the fiery Italian blood that occasionally ran through her veins. Then there was me; I was the man of the house. All the DIY stuff appeared on my to-do list.

We kept the house spotless, never had any arguments, and once a week or so I drove us all to the shops for groceries. We joked about the easy domestic bliss of our self-created family.

My room was on the ground floor, just past the lounge room. It was perfect because I didn't have to stagger up any stairs after a big night out. I had my own washroom further down the corridor on the way to the kitchen, and getting ready in the morning without disturbing the girls was easy.

I had told the girls about my collapsed lung, but so far, so good. Other than the occasional twinge around the scar from the surgery and a couple of weird muscle spasms, it was like the whole thing had become a mere blip on the radar of my life. I slowly built up my fitness with jogging and weights, and my dream of the Himalayas once again seemed within reach.

Bow wasn't the safest suburb in London, but you could get cheap rent, a good curry and, arguably, the best bagels in the world. The most famous historical thing about Bow was that it was walking distance from Whitechapel – the old stomping ground of Jack the Ripper. Our house was kind of famous too. In the 1930s, it had been a nursery school and was visited by the legendary Mahatma Ghandi during his brief stay in East London. According to stories, the kids all called him Uncle Ghandi. It was cool to think that Ghandi might once have sat having tea in our very lounge room.

All in all, life was pretty sweet. A couple of weeks earlier, my work had granted me a scholarship to study at King's College in London, and in November, I was going to start a Master's degree in pain management. I had been lucky enough to have been chosen out of a couple of hundred candidates. The scholarship would save me around twenty thousand dollars. Yes, life was pretty sweet. Within weeks with the girls, we really felt like a family.

I had no idea, but I was soon to need family big time.

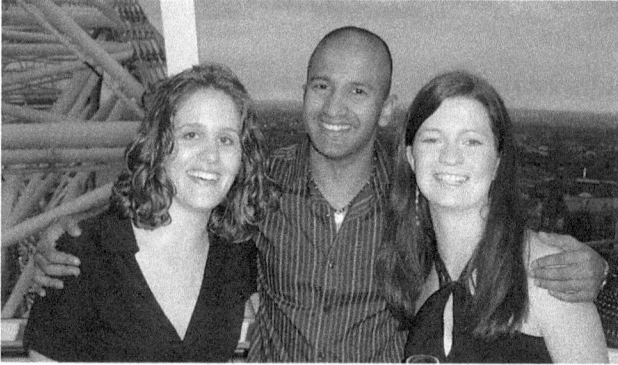

Me with Lauren (left) and Anita (right) at the London Eye

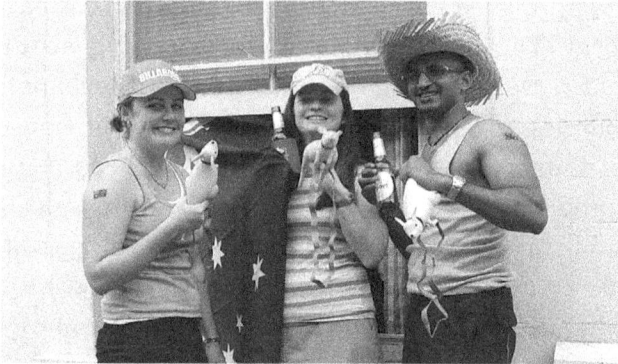

Soccer World Cup fever, from left, Jill, Anita and me

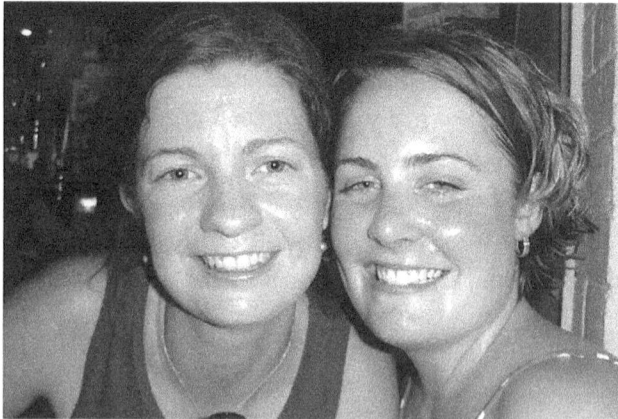

A usual Friday night at home with Anita and Jill (right)

FIREBALL OF DESTINY

I settled into the Bow house with the girls, and that's how I came to be sitting on the couch in our tiny lounge room with Jill on Friday 23 June 2006, watching football, which is soccer if you are an Aussie. The tiny lounge room was at the front of our house. Two couches were squeezed around the TV and a long coffee table.

I was finishing off some chocolate ice-cream straight from the container and Jill was relaxing next to me with a beer. Lauren was leaving to go back to her home in up-state New York and was upstairs packing in her room. Anita was in the kitchen preparing food for the farewell barbeque we had planned for the following day. The girls had it all organised and it was my pleasure to stay right out of their way, eating ice-cream on the couch and watching TV. Not that I was getting out of it lightly; my shift would come later at the cleaning-up stage. They cooked and I cleaned up.

Our small lounge room had one large window that faced out onto the street. Our front yard – if you could even call it that – was concrete, about two meters deep with a waist high wall to separate us from the pavement and the road we lived on. As soon as we turned the light on at night, the blind had to come down because you could see right inside. Because we lived directly opposite a seedy council estate, it was best not to advertise the fact that you had a TV, or anything else for that matter.

Just the day before, riot police broke up a massive gang fight between West Indians and their Bangladeshi rivals from a neighbouring high-rise. Machetes, knives and poles were the weapons of choice for this particular rumble. Word on the street was that it wasn't so much a racial war, but a turf war.

I hadn't been home when it happened, but Jill had watched it peeping through the curtains from upstairs. She had called me and told me to come home, and even though I raced home, it was all over by the time I sped up our street on my motorbike. Jill filled us all in on the drama. She was shaking as she described people being chased by machete-wielding gang members and cops with their riot gear.

We all knew it wasn't the safest of neighbourhoods, but nothing like this had happened before. We weren't really worried, I guess, because when you are not part of the problem, you never imagine that you could get caught up in it. Having grown up in Melbourne during the gangland wars, I and everyone I knew, always felt safe from the violence because of an understanding – true or not – that gangs fought each other and left everyone else alone.

When I came home from work that afternoon, the streets were empty except for some leftover shattered glass and a bit of debris. There was no reason to think that the gangs would fight again on the night after, when Jill and I sat on the couch in front of the TV. Everything seemed peaceful enough, not a police officer in sight. We all felt comforted by the *absence* of any law enforcement that evening, and figured that if the cops suspected there would be another fight, they would have been there.

Jill finished her beer-break and wandered back to the kitchen to help Anita while I finished off the ice-cream. I was on cloud nine because I had just asked a girl I liked to be my girlfriend. Her name was Bhavini – but everyone called her Vin. She was a beautiful free spirit who made me laugh. I think it was her positive energy that I loved most about her. There was so much packed into her tiny 5 foot frame.

Vin and I had known each other for about six months before we actually met. She was a friend of a friend and we became e-pals, then phone pals. I first met her in person when she visited London in 2004. I called her a gremlin on steroids. She never sat still and always wanted to be doing something. *Let's go jet-boating!* or *Let's go to Germany tomorrow!* I never knew what crazy idea she would come up with next, but her energy next to my calm seemed to fit. Time, distance and other relationships got in the way of anything happening back then, and we even lost touch for a while. But she had recently visited again and we just continued where we left off. It was so easy. What's more, this time, the time was right – we were both single and she talked about moving to London to work.

Vin was living in Sydney, but I didn't want to wait. Over the phone, I asked her if she was interested in me. When she said she was, it felt like a piece of the puzzle fell into place. I wanted her energy; I wanted to be the kind of person who could always stay positive, the kind of person who would do things on a whim; I wanted to fight the practical laid-back part of me by basking in the shining light of her. She was the flame. I was the moth.

It was just before 10 pm, when suddenly, there was the sound of glass smashing. Before my mind could fully register the noise, glass from our lounge room window scattered all over the carpet. I looked all around me to see what had come through the window. Was it a ball? Was it a rock? Two youths appeared at the hole where our window used to be. They grabbed the Venetian blind and pulled it outwards, cracking it and leaving it dangling on its hinges.

I had enough time to register surprise and looked on frozen at one of the youths who held a clear glass bottle with a rag poking out of its neck in one hand and a lighter in the other. His face was a shadow as he brought his arms together, uniting flame and wick. The fire caught and the rag flared up.

There was a whooshing sound as he took aim and threw the bottle at me, like pitching a baseball. Only seconds passed and my world turned silent but for my heartbeat: *thump-thump, thump-thump, thump-thump.*

The flame trail illuminated the room with a fiery orange glow

It radiated heat.

Thump-thump.

My arm flew up to deflect the flaming bottle.

Thump-thump.

It smashed against the wall above my head.

Thump-thump.

Glass and a liquid that smells like petrol rained down on me.

Thump-thump.

Heat flared in a whoosh.

Thump-thump.

Fire.

I was on fire.

Flames snaked up the wall behind me and along my arms.

'You got the wrong guy!' I screamed at the youths at the window, not knowing whether they had more bottles of fire to throw at me. But then adrenaline kicked in. 'Help!' I screamed, whacking furiously at my arms and my body to stop the flames. It was like a thousand wasps buzzing that I was trying to keep from stinging me.

Stop-drop-and-roll, immediately came to my mind. But I was in London – *there is never any room to do that, let alone in our tiny lounge room.*

I was trapped because the couch and the walls were on fire, blocking my exit. I ran around the coffee table, crunching over the broken glass on the floor in my bare feet. I leapt over the flames that were crawling across the carpet, and ran through the doorway. I had enough presence of mind to slam the door shut behind me as I fled the burning room. Anita and Jill were running down the hallway, summoned by the smashing sound of glass, and then my screams.

'Get out!' I screamed at them. 'The house is on fire!' I ran into the kitchen towards the tap. Cold water gushed over my arms and I splashed water like a maniac. I felt no pain, but I could see skin peeling off both my arms. My skin looked like moist potato peel. At first I thought it was only my arms, but as feeling returned when my adrenaline rush subsided, I felt a burning behind my left ear and realised that the flames had licked around and burnt me.

The girls rushed past me and out the back door. I was glad they were out, but seconds later, they were back lugging a hose, tugging it towards the hall. I saw it, but I didn't really take it in.

As my thinking started to return, I knew from first aid training that I needed to immerse myself in cold water. As my feeling started to return, I knew I was in trouble. My whole head hurt and felt seared. I fled towards the stairs and ran up to the bathtub. I ran the cold water bath tap, stepped into the bath fully clothed and stood under the shower head. I blasted that too and sat down.

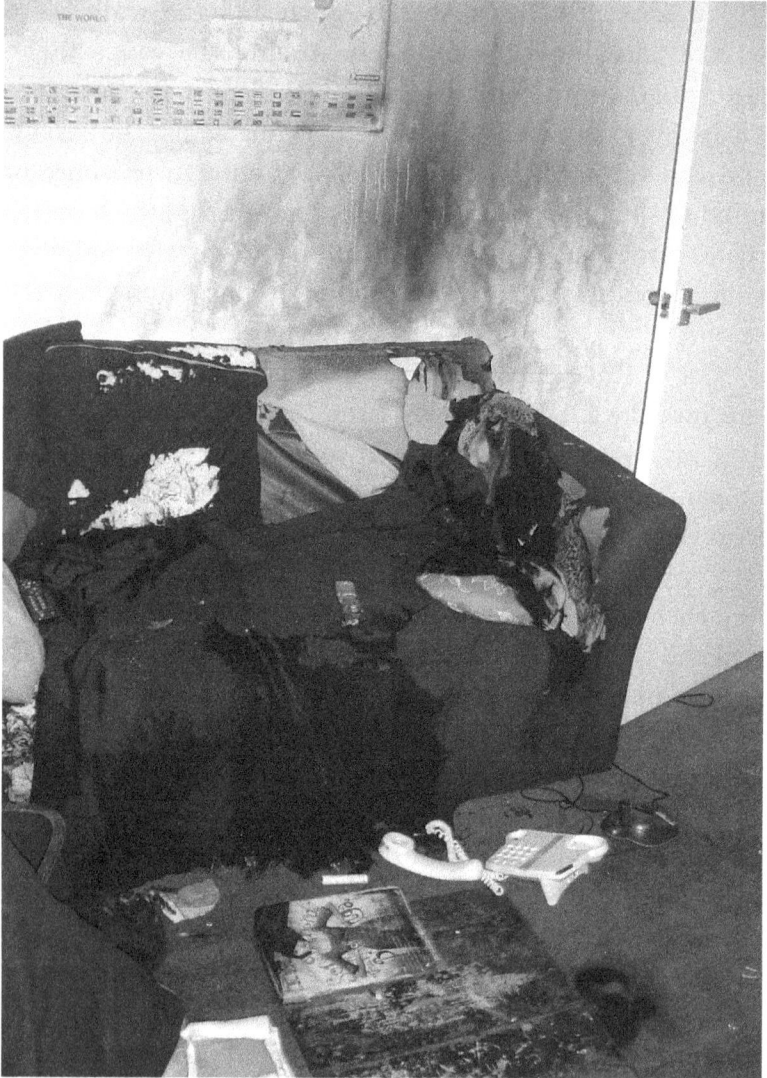

The burnt couch and the black stain where the petrol bomb hit the wall (where my head would have been if I hadn't ducked)

It was like a horror movie. My skin was like wet wrinkled tissues. There was blood everywhere: trailing in lines, trickling from my skinless arms and smeared over the bathroom wall and the bathtub. My left foot stung and I realised that I'd cut it on the broken glass downstairs. From under the freezing shower, I could see outside the bathroom door and I could see smoke and smell the odour of burning fuel. I imagined that the flames must have caught and the whole house was on fire. I could hear the girls yelling downstairs.

I was faced with a choice: should I stay where I am and risk being trapped, or should I flee and guarantee permanent damage to my body? I knew enough about first aid to understand that the cold water preserves the skin and slows inflammation. It stops the air from reacting with the raw skin underneath and alleviates the pain. I decided to risk it and stay in my new cold wet world.

My breath came in quick foggy puffs as fast as my heartbeat. I shivered and froze under the water and imagined this was the end. An eerie sense of peace came over me as I accepted my reality – *this was it.*

I wanted to tell my family that I loved them; I wanted to tell Vin that I really loved her, but that she should move on and find new love; I wanted to see my baby niece one more time; I wanted my family to know that I made a choice to stay in the bath to risk survival. It was not that I wanted to die, because I didn't. I just wanted them to know that I held my own fate in my burnt hands.

After thinking my goodbyes to my family, a surge of survival instinct flooded through me like a golden light, illuminating hope.

Amid the yelling from downstairs, I heard Lauren's voice floating up. She was calling 999. And she was still in the house. Relief flowed over me as I made the connection; if they were still in the house, then the house was not burning down and I might not die.

Ironically, with the relief came pain: searing pain. As feeling returned with a fiery vengeance, the icy water offered scant relief. But pain was not the only thing I needed to deal with. With my life no longer on the line, a floodgate of emotions opened. Thinking of my family made me want to cry with self-pity.

Why is this happening to me?

My lower lip trembled and I almost cried.

Get a grip; it's not over yet.

This was not helping me. My pain was starting to worsen. It occurred to me that what I have learnt about pain was true – pain is more than just damaged tissues. The emotional aspect is just as important.

The theory was now a reality. I could *feel* it. Panic and it gets worse; calm down and it's not quite as bad. I must have been panicking because the pain got worse in such strong waves that just as I thought it couldn't possibly get any stronger, it did.

I forced myself to be calm. Breathe. Slowly. In. And out.

I stared down at my arms. My damaged arms. And my hands. The hands that I needed to heal others.

What was I going to do?

How could I ever work again?

How was I going to explain this to my parents?

Lauren appeared at the door, speaking into the cordless phone. When her eyes looked up and she saw me, she stopped dead in her tracks. Her face looked like she was at a horror movie. She was stone-cold stunned. I realised that I must have looked bad and not only that, but my blood had smeared everywhere when I had struggled with the taps and trying to steady myself under the shower.

'Yes he is already in the shower,' Lauren said frantically to the 999 operator.

'Tell them I'm burnt. Tell them I'm burnt,' I interrupted, shivering under the icy shower.

'He's burnt really bad!' she yelled into the phone.

Suddenly, Lauren backed away from the doorway and was replaced by two fireman dressed in bulky yellow fire suits.

'Get something for my arms! They're burning up!' I yelled at them. Their presence brought me a small sense of relief. The fact that they were up here, meant that the fire mustn't have spread.

One of the firemen yelled down the stairs to someone. Moments later, a third fireman appeared, and handed some towels to the guy closest to me. He placed what looked like over-sized tea towels on both my arms. The cloths were oily with some kind of ointment that had an immediate effect – my arms went from fiery to cool. Or cooler at least.

This has to be a dream. This has to be a dream.

The fireman closest to me, opened a bag and pulled out a gas bottle with a mouthpiece like a snorkel. 'This will help with the pain,' he said. 'Bite on the mouthpiece and breathe in deeply.'

Shivering and shaking, I tried to slow my breathing and calm down a bit. 'I have had a collapsed lung,' I gasped. 'Will this affect it?'

The fireman looked down at the tube and shrugged. 'Not sure,' he said, frowning.

Sod it, I thought. 'Just give it to me.' Anything to reduce the pain. I sucked wildly on the tube and glanced down and saw it wasn't connected to the gas bottle. Without the use of my hands to remove the mouthpiece, I tried to talk with tube still in my mouth to tell them.

'Calm down,' said the fireman, clearly misinterpreting my grunts as distress.

I spat out the tube. 'It's not connected!' I said, wildly. I am normally a mild-mannered sort of guy, but all etiquette flew out the same window the petrol bomb came in through.

The fireman fumbled with the cord and the gas bottle, and finally, I was able to get the gas into my body. It didn't help at all and I spat it out in disgust.

The moist ointment towels had started to dry, and with their drying the burning welled back up again to unbearable proportions. 'It's not working. Get me some more of those towels,' I pleaded.

The fireman lifted off the old towels and replaced them with new ones. 'These are all we've got, mate' he said in a thick East London accent. 'We're gonna have to pull your shirt off,' he said, trying to grasp the bottom of my T-shirt to pull it up.

'No!' I cried, having a vision of my skin coming off with it. 'Just cut it off!' I realised that these guys might not actually know what they were doing. I could feel rather than see him cutting the back of my T-shirt, then the sleeves. I could feel him slowly peeling it away. From the feel of it, I don't think any skin came with it.

He then said that he would need to slide off my watch. 'This might pull off some skin,' he warned.

'Cut the bloody watch off,' I growled.

Behind him, at the doorway, a guy appeared in an ambulance uniform.

'I need to get to a burns unit,' I told him. 'I may have second and third-degree burns.'

The ambulance guy raised his hands in apology. 'I've only come in the car. We'll have to wait for the ambulance to arrive to take you to the hospital.'

What?

These guys weren't helping. My mind raced. I needed to take control. Next of kin. First things first. I called out Uncle Jine's telephone number. If anything happens...

'Calm down, mate,' the fireman said sternly.

'I'm freezing. I'm hyperventilating. I don't know if I'm going to faint so get this down!' I spat out the words. Not only had my manners fled through the window, but I think by this time, they had left Bow.

The fireman patted his pockets for a pen and something to write on. He found the pen, but there was no paper. He looked down at his arm. I repeated the number and he wrote it on his forearm.

'Where's the damn ambulance?'

'It's coming,' the ambulance officer said.

'This is bullshit, guys. I'm burning up.'

Could things get any more ridiculous?

They could.

I swear the ambulance took half an hour. By the time it got there, a policeman had joined the party in the bathroom. He busied himself helping the firemen. From under my curtain of icy water in the shower, I watched the goings-on and listened to their conversation about the logistics of getting me down our narrow stairs.

'We'll try and get a stretcher up here to get you downstairs,' the fireman said once they got word the ambulance had arrived.

My legs weren't burnt, just my head and arms. 'I can walk,' I told them, impatiently. I didn't want to waste any more time; I had to get to the hospital to save my arms. Not waiting for their reply, I struggled to my feet and stood upright.

Problem solved, the men in the bathroom helped me climb out of the bath. Behind me, they turned off the icy shower.

Parts of me were so relieved to get out of the shower, while other parts of me started to well with pain once the cold water stopped flowing over me. With my hands wrapped in towels out in front of me, I walked like a mummy towards the stairs. Spurred on by the waiting ambulance and the thought of being in the Burns Unit, I moved quite quickly down the stairs and straight out the front door. I scanned the crowds and flashing lights outside for the ambulance.

Where the hell was it?

It was just like the movies: people were gathered around; police, ambulance and the fire brigade were present; lights were flashing and people were being asked to stay back. I kept seeing strangers looking at me with sympathy and disbelief.

Once I was out the door, two ambulance officers met me with a wheelchair and carefully sat me in it. The ambulance was parked down the road a bit. I wondered if the youths who did this to me were in the crowd, watching.

Anger welled inside me from a source I didn't understand and couldn't explain. 'Who the hell did this to me?' I screamed at the crowd. I wanted to face them. To make them realise they got the wrong guy. To tell them how stupid they were. To show them I was a human being. To show them what they had done. To shame them.

Tonight was clearly shaping up to be the night that I said all the things I would never normally say, to speak my thoughts out loud. Or yell them, as the case may be.

From the chair to a stretcher, I was loaded into the ambulance.

'Anj!' Anita's face appeared in the double doors.

'Did everyone get out okay?' I asked urgently.

'Yes, we're all fine! What do you want us to do?' Anita was in teacher mode, but there was an underlying panic in her eyes.

'Can you come in the ambulance with me?' If Anita was with me, she could keep the others in the loop.

'She can't come; she's not family,' one of the ambulance officers interrupted.

Anita looked like she was going to argue, but a police officer climbed into the ambulance as the paramedics were closing the doors.

'Get my phone and contact my uncle,' I told her quickly. And then she was gone. Sirens wailed as we sped away.

The policeman sat on a stretcher adjacent to mine.

'Are the girls going to be taken care of?' I asked him, needing to know they were going to be okay.

'They'll be fine; they're getting checked out and then they will meet you at the hospital,' he reassured me.

'Why me?' I asked. 'I haven't done anything wrong.'

The policeman had concern in his eyes. He spoke in a gentle voice. 'It's probably a case of mistaken identity,' he said. 'We think the target was one of your neighbours.'

It suddenly struck me that the house two doors down also had a blue door. I didn't know the people who lived there, so I couldn't make any judgement as to whether they might be more worthy recipients of a fire-bomb attack than me.

'Did you see who did this to you?'

'They looked Bangladeshi,' I said. 'One of them had a T-shirt with horizontal coloured stripes.' While I was answering, I got a flashback to the two guys standing at my broken lounge room window. It was crazy to think that one minute, I had been sitting on the couch eating chocolate ice-cream, and the next, two strangers are throwing a flaming bottle at me. *Why?*

'We had a tip-off,' the policeman said.

'About the attack?'

'We got a tip-off that something would happen around 10 o'clock.'

'There was a huge gang fight with swords and machetes last night. Why weren't there more police around today?' I asked in disbelief.

He shrugged. 'There's nothing we can do if we don't know where it's going to happen. We can't be everywhere at once.' For a moment, he looked helpless.

I understood, but it didn't make my situation any easier on this crazy, crazy night.

FROM HOSPITAL WORKER TO HOSPITAL PATIENT

The word *pain* comes from the Latin name *Poena*, the Greek goddess of revenge, retribution, or penalty. In ancient times, many cultures believed that pain was a punishment for wrongdoing. When the world stopped looking to the gods for answers, modern therapists defined pain as an unpleasant sensory and emotional experience associated with actual or potential tissue damage. While my tissue was certainly damaged, my pain felt more like the old-fashioned kind – the gods had smitten me good and proper.

Despite the lights and sirens of my swift ambulance drive, when we arrived at the hospital, there was no rush to get me into the burns unit. In fact, according the ambulance driver, the hospital didn't even have one.

I was wheeled in through the doors of Accident and Emergency on a stretcher. A nurse asked me for my medical history and personal details. I told them everything I could remember in a hoarse voice. The nurse poked an icy-pole stick into the back of my tongue and made me say ahhhh.

'Your tongue and throat are a bit swollen from smoke inhalation,' she explained. 'That's why you're hoarse.'

I moaned at a particularly savage wave of pain in my arms and hands. 'Whatever you do save my hands! I need my hands for work!' As I tried to stifle the next cry of pain, I thought back to the times I had worked in the Accident and Emergency department. As a staff member, you always hope that your patients are quiet so they don't cause panic among other patients.

'I'm so sorry for whining,' I panted at the nurse. 'It just really hurts.' It was at that moment that I vowed to never underestimate someone else's pain. How often had I stood right where my nurse now stood, at the end of a hospital bed, and not appreciated what the person who lay before me was going through?

After the official stuff was over, they cut through what remained of my jeans and put me in a hospital gown. The scene then changed. Like some strange psychedelic movie, I was pumped full of morphine while people in white uniforms wrapped me in cling wrap. The drugs acted like a curtain between my awareness and my pain. It was still there, but it wasn't the throbbing burning searing entity it had been. I floated happily on a drug-induced cloud.

'My hands are like pappadams,' I giggled, holding up my hands with the bulging cream-coloured flesh.

A young nurse looked up from my chart. 'Your birthday is the same as mine,' she said.

'I look like I'm wearing a human condom,' I told her, grinning.

She smiled at my cling-wrapped body, clearly used to people who had been drugged to the hilt. 'The cling wrap is to stop the air from reacting with your skin,' she explained. 'The nerve endings become very sensitive when they come into contact with air. Because you've lost several layers of skin, your nerve endings are more exposed.'

'I still look like I'm wearing a big condom.'

'Yes, you do,' she conceded. Then her smile faded. 'Your face is pretty burnt.'

'I don't care about my face,' I said. 'Chicks dig scars.' And then it was my turn to be serious. 'Save my hands,' I told her. 'I need them for my work. I'm a physio.'

'Don't worry, we'll look after you.'

I was reassured by her calmness.

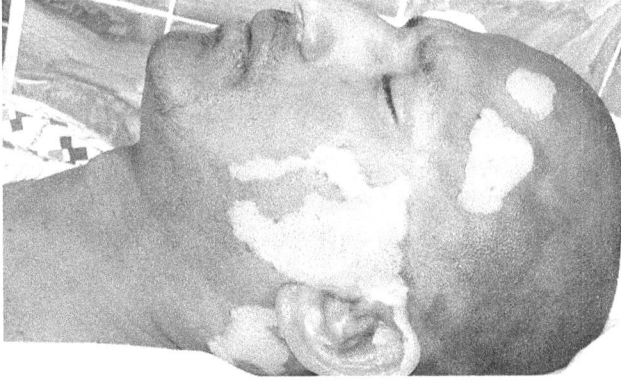

My burnt face

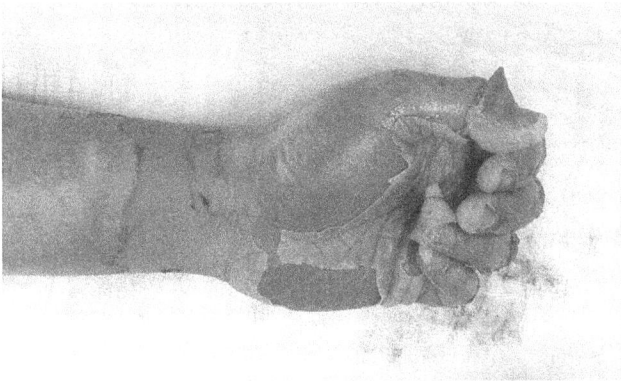

My scorched hand

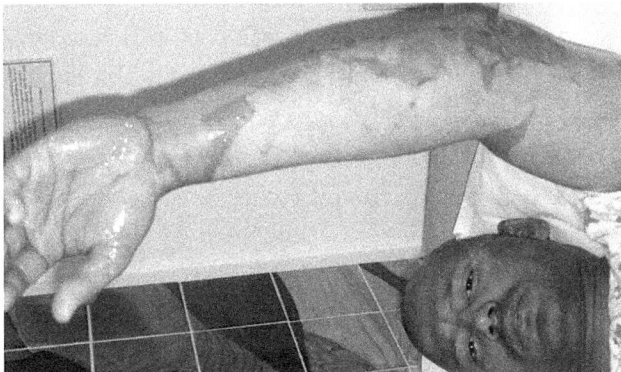

Lying in hospital for hours

Over the next five and half hours, I lay in a cubicle wrapped in cling wrap and connected to an intravenous drip that was periodically injected with morphine. At one point, Anita, Jill and Lauren appeared by my bedside. They looked like triplets of concern. Faces creased with worry. Faces puffy from shock, worry and perhaps tears. Faces frightened for me.

'How funny is this?' I had to try to ease their concern.

They all looked at me with shock.

'Look at the irony. We were getting ready for a barbeque and some moron barbequed me instead!' I laughed hoping that I could make them laugh.

The girls didn't laugh but because I was laughing so hard, eventually, they grinned. Tension released.

'We thought you were on your way to a burns unit,' Jill said.

'The nurse told me that someone had entered the wrong code or something. I'm stuck here till another ambulance is available to take me to a burns unit.'

'What do you mean?' said Jill in utter disgust and disbelief.

'That's outrageous!' said Anita.

'Bloody NHS!' said Lauren.

We were joined by my 22-year-old cousin Nadie, who was more than just a cousin. Over the years we had become close and now she was more like a sister. She'd been out with a friend when Anita had called to tell her what had happened. The girls hugged her and then she came to my bedside. I saw the look of astonishment in her eyes, like she was trying to hide her shock.

Without a mirror, the only way I could judge what I might now look like was in the faces of others. It wasn't looking good.

'We have to stop meeting like this,' she joked. 'You don't have to go to this extent to get attention.'

'Nadie, you know, there is a lesson to be learnt: don't stay home on a Friday night,' I joked. Then I realised with a shock – *Vin*! I had been single so long and it was only tonight that I officially had a girlfriend. 'Can you let Vin know what happened?'

Anita told Nadie and me how the girls had put out the fire and – apart from me – there wasn't a lot of damage beyond the living room. The girls all seemed fine apart from a bit of smoke inhalation. Anita showed me my mobile phone. The outside casing was melted and black. I was lucky the inside was okay and that she could notify my relatives. She put it on the cabinet next to my bed. A little charred reminder of our horrible night.

THE VIEW FROM THE BED

The realisation that I almost died that night really hit me during the ambulance ride to Broomsfield Hospital's burns unit. Friday 23 June could have been my last night on earth, and I was bloody lucky it wasn't. Even though I was badly injured, I was alive.

I knew I had a battle ahead of me, and I also knew that I would do whatever it took to overcome this. I always need to find a purpose in anything that I undertake; when I set my mind to something, I work from dawn till dusk if need be. This new personal challenge would be my next project. This I knew.

Eight months earlier, when I suffered the collapsed lung, I fought my way back. I was in hospital for five weeks and then had life-saving lung surgery. My slow climb back to fitness had taken a full commitment on my behalf. In fact, I had registered for a ten kilometre fun-run to be held in three weeks time. Clearly, that would now have to wait.

By the time I got to Broomsfield Hospital at 6 o'clock the next morning, I knew I was going to fight: fight for me and fight for my future. I also knew that my work in pain management would serve me well. I would just have to practice what I preached.

Again!

First it was the pain of my collapsed lung, and now I had a different kind of pain. But from where I stood – or lay, to be more exact – pain is pain, and no matter how bad or different, I still needed to deal with it.

When my care had been handed over to a nurse at Broomsfield, I went to shake the hand of the nurse who had accompanied me in the ambulance, but I realised that I couldn't. It was awkward. I stuck my hand out and both of us looked down at the cling wrap that couldn't conceal the red and rawness of my burnt hand. I shrugged and withdrew it. I couldn't give her a hug because that would be a bit weird. Instead, I promised to come back and thank her once I was back on my feet.

When the cling wrap was removed during my first examination at the burns unit, I saw huge blisters on my arms and hands that were like large soap bubbles. I'd never seen so many blisters in my life, or ones that were so big. I couldn't believe how much fluid dripped out of my arms. The body releases serous fluid – an inflammatory fluid – to help with the healing process. I had read about it during biology classes at uni, and had actually heard talks about it in pain management. To see first-hand, this clear thick, sticky fluid dripping from me in such quantities that the nurses had to go and get a mop for the floor around me was something very different. It was all over my hospital gown and all over the floor.

I thanked God for my medical knowledge. Without it, I might have found the fluid alarming, but I knew that it was a good sign because it showed that, despite my horrific burns, the healing process in my body had started. I knew that the fluid helped stop the bleeding, clean the area and rid it of dead tissue.

A nurse explained that my wounds would need to be photographed because it was a criminal case. The word *criminal* jolted me. It was so hard to believe that I was a

victim of crime. I suddenly understood the frequent use of
the term *innocent victim* in newspaper and media reports.
I was an innocent victim; I had done absolutely nothing
to provoke the attack on me. From what the cop had said
to me, I might have simply been sitting in the house with
the wrong blue door. Lying there, watching my arms drip
with fluid, the most predominant emotion inside of me was
disbelief. How could something like this happen? It was
surreal.

The morphine drip that had travelled with me from the
Royal London Hospital continued to do its job. I experienced little pain and slept intermittently. I felt like I'd run
a marathon and I hardly registered when the nurse told
me that I had to go to theatre for them to clean up my
wounds. The anaesthetic completed my trip to la-la land.

With my arms bandaged like a mummy, I woke up late
morning in a ward with three other beds, each housing a
burns victim like me. A nurse checked my chart and explained
that I had second- and third-degree burns to my arms, and
superficial burns to my face, head, neck, stomach and left
lower leg.

What?

I tried to flick back the blankets with my unwieldy
bandaged hands to check the rest of me. I had been so
focused on the injuries to my hands and arms that I hadn't
registered burns anywhere else. The nurse saw me struggle
and came around and gently lifted the covers. There was a
fist-sized burn on my stomach. I suddenly became aware of
stinging sensations in all the places she said I was burnt.
Funnily enough, before I knew I had them, I hadn't felt
them at all.

What next? While the drip filled me with replacement
fluids and pain killers, my natural mind-set kicked in.

What's next? What do I have to do to help myself? I asked to see the doctor. I needed answers.

A doctor, whose name I didn't catch, stood by my bed and filled me in on my situation. He flipped open my chart and read it. 'We are giving you anti-inflammatory pain medication,' he explained, nodding towards my drip. 'You'll probably have the medication for about ten days until we're sure that there are no further complications or infections.'

'Why ten days?' I asked.

'The inflammatory stage only lasts ten days,' said the doctor. 'Unless there are complications, anti-inflammatory medications won't really have any effect after that.'

A connection sparked in my mind. All the stuff I'd been doing with patients in pain management now applied to me. I knew I needed physio, but I would need a physiotherapist who was an expert in burns. I knew that the sooner I started, the better it would be for my hands. A couple of days after you get an injury, like a little cut, you begin to feel a little bump under the skin. The bump is formed by the collagen in the tissue ends joining up to bind the edges of a wound together, and then it shrinks to really hold it in place tightly. We physios call it the contraction stage. I knew from my training that if the collagen is allowed to shrink too much, the scar tissue becomes tight. This is why physio was so important for me. As my skin started to form scar tissue from the burns, it would tighten. That meant I would have a daily program of stretches and gentle exercise ahead of me. I was keen to start.

'When is the physio going to see me?' I asked with eagerness.

'Settle down,' said the doctor, grinning. 'First things first. You need to rest up for a bit. You've just come out of surgery.'

I relaxed back into my pillows. He had a point. My body had just been through a massive shock and I did feel a little tired. I could get fired up about my treatment... Tomorrow.

As I woke from a doze when someone called my name, I blinked and registered my surroundings. Bandages. Burnt. Hospital. The nurse.

'Anjelo, you've got a phone call,' she said gently. 'It's your dad.'

Oh no. What was I going to say to him?

I struggled out of bed and pushed the pole with my IV drip along in front of me as I followed the nurse to the nurses' station. She helped as I fumbled with the receiver, trying to wedge it under my chin because I had mummy-hands. 'Hello...' I said tentatively, waiting for it.

'How are you? Are you okay? Are you going to sell your motorbike now?' Dad fired questions like bullets.

Huh? 'What's my motorbike got to do with anything?' I stammered.

'We're coming to look after you!'

I had visions of my parents rushing onto a plane, Mum hysterical and crying all the way from Melbourne to London, them both running to my bedside and smiling at me then bursting into tears.... Again! They have done this already when I was in hospital the last time with a collapsed lung. I didn't even have to imagine the scenario because I'd seen it already. In their eyes, I would go from being their 28-year-old son to their helpless baby boy. Mum would fuss and try to feed me. Extreme parenting – they would love it, but my reputation, my street-cred, would be in tatters. I got this immediate vision of me lying on my bed, being macho for some visiting friends: *Yeah, I survived a petrol bomb*, I would say suavely, and then my mum would interrupt with a spoonful of jelly flying like an aeroplane towards my mouth. *Just one more mouthful.*

Yep, kiss the street-cred goodbye.

'No... you don't need to come. Seriously, I'll be okay. I am already walking around.' I tried to sound healthy and convincing.

'We're coming,' he declared. 'We've already bought the tickets.'

Bugger!

'I'm at the nurses' station,' I told Dad. 'I probably need to get off the phone.' I suddenly needed to lie down. It's all very well to be strong for strangers, but in the tsunami of emotions that accompanies my parents whenever one of their children is sick, it's hard to remain strong. Their concern is kind of catching. I pictured their worry, which I knew would then make me worry. But I loved them for it, even if sometimes they drove me a little crazy.

It was a nurse who helped feed me when lunch arrived – more preferable to Mum. The only thing I was able to do for myself was clamp a cup between my bandaged palms and drink through a straw. Even without Mum there, I quickly realised that I needed help with toileting, showering, dressing, eating and cleaning my teeth – so I had to be treated like a baby anyway.

I'd just finished lunch when my cousin Nadie appeared at my bedside along with Uncle Jine and Aunty Mal. Again. How many times had they visited me in hospital? Uncle Jine is known to worry at times. While he spoke really quickly – *You'll be fine, you'll be fine, this is a good hospital, they'll look after you well here, it looks new* – I could tell from the worry in his eyes that he was trying to convince me and himself that things would be okay. He then checked my chart and nodded enthusiastically over the list of drugs I had been given.

Ying to his yang, Aunty Mal was calm and softly spoken, almost hypnotic. 'We've spoken to your parents,' she said gently. 'Is there anything else we can do for you?'

It was deja vu. Their presence – again at my hospital bedside – made me feel guilty. They had been amazingly supportive when I had the collapsed lung. Now they were back to support me again. 'I'm so sorry I've done this to you again–'

'Don't be silly!' my uncle interrupted. 'You are family!'

'There's no need to apologise,' said Aunty Mal in her smooth voice. 'You did nothing to cause this. We'll always be there for you.'

I could only mutter my thanks, and then words failed me. Aunty Mal was right. I did nothing to provoke what had happened. It wasn't my fault. I didn't understand it any more than they did.

As much as I couldn't explain why, I could certainly explain the rest, telling them step-by-step what had happened last night. In a rush, I told them my surreal story... *I was sitting on the couch... next thing, guys smash our window... flaming petrol bomb... I was on fire... there wasn't enough room to stop-drop–'n'-roll... my skin peeled off.*

To their credit, my shocked aunt and uncle stood without expression, listening to my night of horror. After keeping their visit short, they left their shopping bags of biscuits, chocolates and fruit and vanished. I felt exhausted.

Again, I slept.

A single fluorescent light illuminated the far end of the ward that night, casting the rest in dark shadows. I drifted in and out of sleep. The quiet was disturbed in the street two floors below the ward by sudden shouts and voices loud enough for me to hear. Drunken guys maybe. I was suddenly on full alert. And then they did something that frightened me and made me fear for my life – it was the noise of an aluminium drink can being kicked. I held my breath, waiting for another petrol bomb to come through the window. My heart beat in my chest. While my mind knew I was in a safe place, something deeper, more primal, knew that before last night, my lounge room had been safe too. It was at that moment that I realised my injuries weren't just physical, I also suffered a psychological reaction to what had happened. That meant that in conjunction with working on my body, I knew I would also have to work on my mind.

It was a sleepless night.

By Sunday morning, I was feeling sorry for myself. My boss, Vicky, and another colleague appeared by my bedside around 10 am. The can-kicking the night before had made me realise that I had a long road ahead to recovery.

I looked straight into Vicky's eyes. 'I'm so sorry. It wasn't my fault. All I was doing was watching TV at home.' Tears rolled down my cheeks without my permission. Suddenly, it was all too much. The fact that I couldn't go to work was also a hard burden for me to bear. I had only started working with her a year ago.

I believe that you should earn your worth and give one hundred per cent at work. And here I was – for a second time – lying in a hospital bed. I felt guilty for taking so much sick-leave. The tears of frustration came from the fact that I hadn't done anything to contribute to these things. I was just minding my business when fate decided to king hit me again.

Vicky patted the bandage that covered my hand. 'Don't be stupid! This is not your fault. We are just glad that you are okay.'

I calmed myself down and wiped my tears away with

my bandages. With a deep breath, I resumed being me – the normal me, not the bawling me.

After Vicky left, one of my Aussie friends, Duncan, came to visit with his girlfriend Catherine. He and I had been dubbed 'the dynamic duo' at work. We were known for our sarcastic Aussie sense of humour. We were the only two blokes working with about twelve women. We needed to stick together.

Duncan whipped something out of his pocket and held it up in front of me. It was a small fire extinguisher with candy inside it. 'Thought this might help next time,' he said with a smile.

'Bloody bastard,' I muttered.

Then we both burst out laughing.

THE FIRST TIME I SAW YOUR FACE

On Monday, I saw my face for the first time. My new face. My burnt face. It was in a mirror by my bedside, which I hadn't noticed all this while. *Scarface* – that was the first word that came to mind. *Phantom of the Opera*. I had skin peeling along the left side of my face, my left ear looked like a dog had chewed it and my eyelashes were singed. Seeing myself like this, I smelt the petrol – partly in my mind and partly because there was some still on me. My head and scalp were black like charcoal and the back of my neck felt like it had really bad sunburn.

Until that moment, I hadn't given much thought to my face, but looking at the burnt stranger staring back at me from the mirror, I realised I might be scarred for life. *Chicks dig scars*, I reminded myself flippantly. Nonetheless, you take it for granted that your face looks a certain way. It's weird to look in the mirror and see that it has changed – maybe permanently.

Not that scars would really make any difference to me. I had never in my life picked up a girl – that wasn't my style. The few girls I've gone out with in my twenty-eight years of life were all girls that I had befriended first. For me, romance has always come from friendship and not my looks. Vin was no exception. But I didn't want her to be put in a position where she felt obligated to be with me, despite the scars I was sure to end up with.

In one of the few private moments you get in a hospital bed, I struggled for my phone using a combination of bandaged hands and my chin. Feeling like a complete idiot, I reached with my mouth for a plastic pen lid on my bedside table. I bit down hard on it and positioned it so I could push the texting buttons with it. I typed out *call me.*

Within minutes my mobile rang and I pressed the answer button with the pen lid then spat out the lid so I could speak.

'Anj. What's going on?' Vin's rapid-fire conversation held hints of worry. 'Are you okay? Nadie has been keeping me updated. I looked up about burns on the internet. You'll be fine. Don't worry.' Vin paused for breath. Her words were designed to reassure me, but they sounded like they were also reassuring her.

'Vin, I'm okay,' I said, cradling the phone between my bandaged hands. 'Don't worry – that's not what I'm calling about. Um...' I searched for the right words to let her out of her commitment to me. 'Listen, um, maybe it's best that we just stay friends.' My voice quivered. I was doing this for her, not me.

'What! What are you talking about?' She sounded completely shocked.

'I've just seen my face, Vin. It's pretty bad and it's not fair on you. I might be like this forever–'

'Anj, you were ugly before! Lucky I'm not after you for your looks,' she laughed, completely shattering the tense moment.

I was speechless. She was a keeper.

My first physio session happened on that Monday. I watched with interest. By this stage, the bandages had been removed from my hands revealing a synthetic clear film underneath that would simulate my skin until it grew back. It was like a snake skin and the doctor said it would peel off as soon as my new skin appeared.

The physio provided me with exercises. I felt like a kid doing 'Twinkle, Twinkle Little Star', stretching and wriggling my fingers. I had been very conscious of mobility and I'd been wriggling my fingers ever since they were unwrapped. A scorched sensation, like an army of fire ants, ran through my arms. Painfully, I tried to touch my thumb to each of my finger tips in turn. Stretching my skin felt like a band-aid being ripped off. Nonetheless, I knew that the more I did it, the more my body would get used to it and the less it would eventually hurt. Use it or lose it.

How often had I told my patients that to manage pain, you need to address it from both the physical and emotional points of view? It's a natural reaction to stop activity when you experience an injury or have chronic pain. If you twist your ankle, the last thing you want to do is walk on it. But after a short period of rest and an ice-pack treatment, the best thing is to gradually start moving it and putting weight on it, even if it doesn't feel like the right thing to do. If you don't, muscles and ligaments can weaken. On the other hand, if you try too hard or do too much, you don't give your body the chance to recover and heal. I understood how important it was to strike a balance by pacing and grading my activity levels – just like I always told my patients.

Chronic pain also affects us on an emotional level. If you have your activities impeded by their pain, you can suffer from anger, depression and anxiety. Feeling this way often leads to decreased activity resulting in an unhealthy, vicious cycle of pain and disability.

Now, I had to practise what I had been preaching. I looked at this as a sort of test; this was my best chance to prove that the methods that I had been teaching to clients really worked. In the year that I had been working in pain management, I had seen success in the people who applied these principles, and a lack of progress in people who didn't. The biggest difference was in the people who viewed their chronic pain as their identity, as opposed to the people who had a purpose and accepted that they had pain, and were determined to manage it and get on with their lives. A simple distinction but a crucial one in the success or otherwise of dealing with pain.

Two cases I remembered in particular. Emily had chronic back pain since her early teens and by the time she stepped through the door of the pain clinic, she was twenty-six and desperate for relief. She had tried everything to no avail, but that didn't stop her from continuing to seek a solution. She embraced the program with all of her energy and enthusiasm. Her goal was to wear high heels. Not only did she complete all the activities in the right amounts, she also changed her thinking. She began to believe that wearing high heels was a possibility and that self-belief changed everything. What struck me about Emily is that she tried everything with a helpful mind-set and a purpose. At the conclusion of the four-week course, Emily's confidence had grown tremendously, her pain had less impact on her life, and most importantly, she bought a pair of nice high heels and practised and practised until she was able to walk in them.

The second case involved a guy named John. He was middle-aged and had back and arm pain from a lifting injury. He too had tried a lot of different strategies, but the minute John walked in the door, he made it clear that nothing had worked and nothing would work. Any small gains that he made, he dismissed as insignificant. He owned his pain, and his pain owned him. Neither was letting the other go.

So while Emily strode out in her brown high heels, John

and his pain left us unchanged: Emily a shining success, and John a cautionary tale.

From all I had seen, I knew that this process began in my own mind. My thinking was the first thing that I brought to my healing. I knew profoundly that if I implemented the right strategies in the right amounts and believed in the process, it would work. I had to accept that I may have scars for life and that I may end up with chronic pain, but I also had to accept that the kind of life I had was up to me.

I did have one reservation about my new appearance. If my face didn't properly heal, would it interfere with the work that I was so passionate about? In darker moments, I pictured myself sitting in front of the small group sessions that I ran. In this picture, my clients were all gaping at me, looking at my scarred face. But most disturbing was that while they were horrified with my appearance, they weren't listening to my message. This really worried me until I figured out that if my scars didn't heal, then I would use them to my advantage. I could be the example that I would present to my clients:

> *Look at me – look what I went through, but I have learned to manage my pain and my scars. Yes, I accept that my life may never be the same. Yes it's not easy sometimes, but I have not let it stop me and I'm still living my life with a purpose. I practise what I preach. If I can do it, so can you.*

BAD THINGS BRING GOOD PEOPLE TOGETHER

Although I was far from London, most of my friends visited me during those first couple of days in the burns unit. My housemates came in every day, all the way from London. They brought me clothes and anything else that I needed. Jill had gone through my undies drawer and decided that the pairs I had were too old. She went shopping and bought me half a dozen new pairs. With hospitals, you leave your dignity at the door.

Despite disparaging remarks about my undies, the girls kept me company and gave me regular updates on life at home. Lauren had flown back to the States, but Jill and Anita were still at the house. They had nowhere else to go at such short notice. The council had boarded up the front window, and the girls had spent days cleaning up the house with the help of some mates. The burnt couch was carried out for the hard rubbish collection. It was a constant reminder to them of what had happened. I couldn't believe how brave they were to stay there.

Apart from my family and friends, I also had an unexpected visitor. On the third day of my stay in the burns unit, a policeman appeared at the foot of my bed. He had come to take an official statement. We slowly walked to a sitting room for some privacy. Resting awkwardly on an old vinyl couch, I told him what happened. Tears ran down my damaged cheeks.

What's going on here?

I raised my bandaged forearms, and quickly wiped the tears away.

'If we catch 'em, we're going to charge them with attempted murder,' the policeman told me in a sympathetic voice.

Attempted Murder. Instant reality check – someone had tried to *kill* me. The law said so.

'Who were they trying to get,' I asked, wondering what someone could have possibly done to warrant what had happened to me.

'We think it was one of the boys living two doors down. The irony is that he wasn't even home at the time. His mum and 8-year-old sister were sitting in their lounge room when you got attacked in yours.'

The cop at the scene had said the same thing. The teenagers with the Molotov cocktail had mistaken our house for one further down. In moments of self-pity over the last couple of days, I had thought *if only they had got the right house...* Suddenly that thought ceased to exist. Now, I knew what would have happened if they had got the right house. It could have been an 8-year-old girl and her mother on fire. As much as I wished it hadn't been me, I would rather it be me than them.

It was a blessing having so many people who cared about me. The others in my ward weren't so lucky. I shared my section in the burns unit with three other patients. Opposite me was an English guy with a distinctive Essex accent. He was a lean, rough-looking bloke with the physique of a boxer. He was from a place not too far from where I lived. He told me that he got his burns during a nasty argument with his ex-girlfriend; he turned his back on her, and she threw a saucepan full of boiling water at him. I didn't think I had lived a particularly sheltered upbringing, but his story sounded like something that I thought only happened on TV soapies.

'Fooken pathetic, innit?' he declared, as he finished his story.

'Harsh, mate, harsh,' I said, shaking my head in wonder. My story too might sound like something that would only happen on TV: an innocent Aussie physio sitting on his couch eating ice-cream one minute, and on fire from a gangland Molotov cocktail the next. A victim of gang crime. Yep, the more I thought about it, the more my story sounded like a TV plot too.

Next to him and diagonally opposite me was an elderly English gentleman who looked like he might have stepped straight out of an Enid Blyton novel. With his snowy frizzled hair and his rosy cheeks, he looked like he would be at home in an over-stuffed armchair, reading a book and smoking a pipe. But instead, he was here with us. His story really touched my heart. Despite his age, he laboured looking after his three disabled sons who were all in their forties. They lived in his small flat and he told me about how he had converted his living room into a bedroom to fit them all in. He and his wife were devoted parents to their sons, but a year earlier, she had passed away. Every day he lit a candle in her memory and sat it on their coffee table. One night, as he turned to gather some papers and magazines off the floor, he accidentally brushed against the candle flame and his pyjamas caught alight. His burns were mainly on his buttocks and back.

All he was concerned about was his sons – they had been placed in a nursing home while he was in hospital. I had never seen him happier than the day one of the occupational therapists offered to take him to visit his sons.

'I get to see my sons today,' he said, so excited that his eyes filled with tears. He dressed in his old-man's clothes:

pants pulled up way too high, a neat vest, jacket and a tweed hat. Dressed in his Sunday best, he shuffled off beaming.

That night, he told us all about the visit. His sons were happy and the place they were in was nice. Other nights, he tossed and turned in bed, but that night, he slept like a lamb.

I hoped that I'd be half the man he was if I reached his age.

To my left was a man with an extraordinary story of survival. He was a curly-haired young Iranian pharmacist whose father had paid ten thousand dollars to get him out of Iran. He spoke limited English, but using what little he had and the expression in his deep hazel eyes, he told me that he was put in a big car in a hidden smuggler's compartment and had to travel days across the desert. The nights were very cold and the days were very, very hot. At one of the borders, he was transferred into the engine compartment of a bus. The engine had overheated and he had been burnt as a result. Luckily, he was treated soon after, and while his burns were extensive, they weren't too deep. With tears in his eyes, he told me he thought he was going to die.

I could only imagine the guy's horror. It struck me that, when I wanted to come to the UK, I simply saved up and bought a ticket. Here was a guy who was about my age, just as educated as me, yet he had to get smuggled here in a near-lethal engine compartment. It was simply beyond belief.

Even though he now found himself in the UK with no money, clothes or family, he kept saying how grateful he was to be here.

'So where do you go from here?' I asked him, almost dreading the answer.

'The police station,' he replied. 'I will seek asylum here.'

I felt for him because I knew he had a tough road ahead. I called Anita and asked her to bring my track pants and some tops next time she visited. When she brought them in, I walked over to the Iranian's bed and handed them to him.

'Mate you need these more than me,' I said. I also gave him some of the money I had in my wallet.

The guy thanked me about a hundred times.

The burns unit also had children. Further down, there were two little boys who had been burnt when their father added petrol to the family barbecue fire. A freak wind had caught the petrol as he doused the barbecue, making it spray back on the sons who were standing close by. Flames had burst from the fire, and the two sons had caught alight. Another patient was a little girl whose dress caught fire. When she had tried to put it out, she burnt her arms and legs. Another boy, aged about seven, was electrocuted while walking along the street. He had been fishing at a nearby stream, and on the way home, with his fishing rod resting against his shoulder, he crossed a railway line. The rod came in contact with a live overhead electrical wire and the little boy suffered burns to 95% of his body. Even though he was alive, I had never heard of anyone suffering burns to that extent and surviving.

In the burns unit, there were people from many different backgrounds, all with different stories and all brought together by being burnt. During my week there, I learnt something important. No matter how bad things seem, you can always look in a hospital bed nearby and see someone worse off than you. Just when self-pity threatened, I saw or heard of someone who had a lot more cause for self-pity than me. And then, of course, it would be selfish of me to whinge about my situation in the face of those worse off.

That's not to say that there was anything wrong with me declaring that what had happened to me was horrible and that I didn't deserve it. Dwelling on these kinds of thoughts wouldn't serve me though.

It made me appreciate how lucky I was. I was blessed with friends and family who cared for me, and I was blessed with the life I have lived so far.

THINKING ABOUT HEALING

It is not what happens to you that counts, but rather how you deal with it afterwards. Imagine, watching your team win the Grand Final. At the final siren, the winning players jump for joy, laugh and hug each other while doing laps of honour. Compare them with the losing side whose players are exhausted and defeated. Both sides played in the same game and the players are equally exhausted, yet there are two very different physical responses. The final siren brought about two very different consequences for the players from the two teams and it was the thoughts in their minds that brought about their responses, not the game itself.

In the aftermath of the attack on me, the things I'd read about and studied became very real. The event, I couldn't change. It had happened. What I could control were my thoughts and behaviour in the event's aftermath. If I followed the proper path, the consequences for me would be better. I just had to navigate the canyon between *knowing* and *doing*.

The basic theory went something like this: if I was active, I would feel better; if I felt empowered in my own healing, I would feel better; if I had helpful thoughts and a positive mindset, I would feel better.

And of course, if I felt better, I could live life with a purpose. I would do more and be more likely to continue along the road to recovery. I also knew that when I felt better, my body would release adrenaline and endorphins that would increase my feeling of well-being and actually reduce the pain. It's like when you go to the gym and get an endorphin rush, you can't wait to go back because it feels good.

I knew that a positive mindset was helpful and important in healing, but I also knew that the *positive thinking* had to be *helpful thinking*. Every clinician has patients who use positive thinking in unhelpful ways. These patients push through their pain because they are busy thinking positively, but in the end, their recovery periods may be longer, or their pain greater, because they pushed themselves too hard. In pain management, positive thinking can be a double-edged sword.

When dealing with clients, we always explain that a positive attitude is a must, but the accompanying thoughts and behaviour should be *helpful*. I had a client once whose name was Mary. She kept telling me how positive her attitude was, but then she would describe her week and it was anything but positive. She would push through her pain and do the shopping. Then she would have to rest for the remainder of the day because her pain became un-bearable. *Then the house needed cleaning*, she would say, *and so I got up and vacuumed the whole place. Of course, I couldn't move for three days afterwards – but I'm staying positive!*

What Mary was actually doing was positively ruining her chances of a better life because her behaviour and thinking were not helpful – despite her positive attitude.

I wanted to avoid the mistakes that I'd seen my clients make. Right from the start, I had a positive attitude because I made a vow that I would do everything necessary to regain use of my hands and get back to work as soon as possible.

For me, being positive and having helpful thoughts was about knowing my limits and reflecting on what would help and what wouldn't. I had to resist the urge to be the bull in the china shop.

Likewise, if I lay around feeling sorry for myself, or scared to move because of my injuries, it would have the opposite effect. I would fatigue more quickly because my body would de-condition; my muscles and ligaments would tighten, my joints would become stiff, and I would feel lethargic.

One thing I did know is that often people with chronic pain experience increased pain when they are in an unhappy frame of mind. It always came back to my mind: helpful thoughts and a positive mindset. Now I had to practise what I preached.

So from my hospital bed, I did my 'Twinkle Twinkle Little Star' hand exercises, stretched and exercised when I could, followed doctors' orders, and imagined myself at the end of the journey, healed.

After a week in the burns unit, I was discharged into the care of Anita and Jill who were excited to be taking me home. Part of me was thrilled to be getting out of hospital and being with the girls again, but a tiny part of me was nervous about seeing the house. The girls had told me that the walls had been repainted by the landlord and the window was fixed. New carpets had been laid, and because we rented the flat furnished, the landlord had also replaced the couches and the coffee table.

I expected some anxiety and I was curious to see how I would react. The closer we got to Bow and our flat with the blue door, the more a feeling welled up inside me. My senses were hyper-vigilant. We turned into the quiet street, and suddenly the quiet turned into an eeriness. My eyes darted left and right, looking around nervously in case there were boys with Molotov cocktails.

'Holy crap!' I blurted, when I saw the burnt couch outside our place, still waiting for the council pick-up. There was an Anjelo-sized burn silhouette in the centre of one of the seats. I shivered in silence, in horror.

My legs told me to run, but my mind told me that I had to face things. My mind won. Just. The girls carried my stuff inside, leaving me free to make the slow walk from the car to our blue door. The flat looked remarkably the same. Ordinary. As if what had happened, hadn't happened at all. If only I could be fixed so easily.

Rather than smell burnt, our flat smelt like paint and new carpet. That helped. With a deep breath, I stepped into the lounge room. My eyes darted to the window. The blind that the assailants had pulled and bent outwards had been replaced by a crisp white curtain. It was like walking into a different room. All traces of the fire and the attack had been wiped clean in the week I was in hospital. It was a strange cleanliness because the brand new lounge room looked artificial and out of place in the old house.

I sat down on the couch, but then realised that I was in the same place that I was last week and scooted across to a different position. My heart pounded and I couldn't take my eyes off the window. I felt a cold shiver run through my body. My hair would have stood on end, if I had any left. Clinically, I understood my reaction, and was a little bit pleased that I had predicted my response.

In one way, these responses were my body's way of asking me: *Is this a safe place? Should you be here?* The responses were also completely normal, and that in itself was comforting in a weird way. My heart pounding was pumping blood to my legs in case I needed to run. A slight trembling was my body's way of firing my muscles in case

I need to move away quickly. My quickened breathing rate increased my oxygen flow, again to prepare me for a flight response. These responses were primal and kind of fascinating, once I stopped being shit-scared.

I used self-talk – silent self-talk so I didn't look like I'd gone mental – to calm myself. *Slow your breathing. Calm down. You're safe. Everything's fine. This is expected. Breathe in. Breathe out. Slowly. Calmly.*

After several intense minutes of effort, I became calmer.

'Who the hell said I was on the menu for our barbecue?' I asked to lighten the mood.

We all laughed.

My bedroom was heaped with everything that had been salvaged from the lounge room. Magazines, the iron, as well as the DVD and video collection were tossed around like the bomb had hit my room as well. My clothes were strewn everywhere from when the girls had tried to find things to bring into hospital. Normally I'm neat – I'm the kind of guy who makes his bed every morning, and washes and irons his clothes every weekend. I looked at the mess, considered my bandaged hands, and shrugged. It would all have to wait.

'Sorry Anj!' said Anita from behind me. 'It was the only place we could put stuff when they re-did the lounge room.'

'Don't worry about it,' I grinned. The girls had been so amazing that a little mess in my room didn't even register.

Anita and Jill were happy I was home. Our little family was back together again. They fussed around me like nurses. Part of the freaky aftermath of my injury was the peeling skin. That night, using tweezers, Anita attacked my face and head and helped rid me of the peeling bits. It looked as if my left ear was crumbling. Jill helped by packing pillows around me as I tried to get comfortable. They also helped with my arm bandages. My feelings towards these genuine friends deepened with their care. Not only had they been regular cheerful visitors in the hospital, they were prepared to go that extra mile now that I was home.

When we sat around, that first night, it was in the kitchen, not the lounge room. I noticed, without comment, a cautiousness in Jill and Anita. They weren't quite jumpy, but there was an awareness that their home had been invaded and that their safety couldn't be taken for granted.

By unspoken agreement, we didn't talk about how we were feeling. We were just so pleased to be back together again and we all tried to keep our conversational banter upbeat and jokey. Aside from my bandages, we were just like we always were, only now we were pretending that everything was back to normal.

I stayed one night at the Bow house before the girls dropped me at my uncle's to recuperate. I had overwhelming feelings of shame that I was abandoning the girls *again* – leaving them in the house that had been attacked. I promised to keep in contact daily.

Aunty Mal and Uncle Jine offered to have me and I agreed it was the best thing. Not only did they have enough room for me to stay, but they also had enough room for my parents who were, at that moment, sitting in economy somewhere over the Indian Ocean having settled for a crazy route so that they could get to me as soon as they could. I could picture Mum fidgeting, nervous and anxious to get to me. Dad would be calm, hoping it would rub off on Mum, but it usually didn't.

When Mum and Dad arrived the following day, Uncle Jine drove to Heathrow to get them. I wasn't up to travelling yet. Since the attack, my days had involved lots of resting and moderate activity. But activity both exhausted me and hurt me. My burns stung like really bad sunburn all the time and it was worse when I moved or stretched. I absolutely understood how people in my position could curl up and not do anything because that was what my body was telling me to do. However, I knew that wouldn't help me in the long run – what would help was if I could pace my activity so that I gradually built up my strength and endurance. *Gradually* was the key word.

From upstairs in my guest bedroom, I heard the car drive up and the doors opening and closing. This was soon followed by the sounds of the front door and Mum and Dad talking and laughing with my uncle. I had thought of how I would face them. My mum and dad were worrywarts and it was really important that I put on a positive face – even though it was a slightly charred one. At the top of the stairs, I breathed in deeply and set my face into a grin.

Creaking stairs announced me. Mum and Dad both looked upwards. I watched their faces – shock quickly watered down with tentative encouraging smiles. It occurred to me, that right at that moment, my parents and I were doing the same thing – putting on a brave face to hide the enormity of what had happened. I shield them and they shield me right back. This reciprocal shielding is what family is all about.

'Son!' Mum said, relieved. She went to envelop me in a hug and then stopped short, staring in confusion at my bandages and my injuries as if weighing up where she could hug me. Clearly, she decided there was nowhere to hug and patted me awkwardly on the back.

'I'm okay, I'm okay!' I announced. 'It looks worse than it is.' I waved my arms in and out showing them my range of motion.

Dad appeared on the other side of me and kissed me on the cheek. 'We're here to look after you,' he said in his quiet, reassuring way.

Lucky me.

Settled in my aunt and uncle's house in the beautiful open family room that overlooked their tranquil back garden, Mum chatted about the flight. Dad added funny details about Mum on the flight – how she couldn't work the TV controls, and how she ordered the wrong meal – and we all laughed and enjoyed each other's company.

They didn't ask about the attack and I didn't volunteer the story of how I had sat innocently on the couch and the window had been smashed by two dark-clad Bangladeshi teenagers and I had been set on fire in a vicious attack. Not a chance.

It was the same with Jill and Anita – we hadn't talked about it and we tried to be happy for each other. Now Mum, Dad and I were going to do the same thing.

They say confession is good for the soul, but for now, suppression was good for all of our souls. It would be more than two months before I realised how damaging this way of dealing with a trauma could be.

That night I had my first nightmare. I was back at the Bow house, on fire and trying to get out.

RIDING THE ROLLERCOASTER

One night, about two weeks after the attack, my friend Chan came and picked me up for a night out that I badly needed. Before the attack, I rarely spent a night in. Movies, pubs, friends – that was me. Not that I was a party animal, but London was the place to be and I think every young Aussie who lands there makes full use of the nightlife. Mum and Aunty Mal spent most evenings in the kitchen with my cousin Sajith who was an amazing cook. Together they all cooked up a storm. In the lounge room, Uncle Jine and Dad watched a tag-team of CNN and BBC news. It felt like if life went any slower, it would be going backwards. Cabin fever well and truly set in.

They say that in life you need three simple things: someone to love, something to do and something to look forward to. I certainly had people to love and who loved me back, and I had things to look forward to, but I suffered greatly from having nothing to do.

My exercises took fifteen minutes twice a day. Aside from that, I had nothing else to occupy my up-until-now active mind. Mum and Dad helped clean my wounds twice a day and I felt like a baby – a bored helpless cranky baby. I couldn't believe that I had left Melbourne to be more in-dependent, yet here I was dependent on my parents for almost every need. They even had to feed me because I didn't have the dexterity to pick up a fork.

Deep down I knew that this was an irrational way of thinking because I had undergone a major trauma and needed all the help I could get; but I just wanted to get back on my feet.

I was grateful when Chan came to rescue me from my boredom. He arrived at my aunty and uncle's house and, even though I wanted to grab him and run out the door to the freedom of a night out, Chan wandered in, chatted to my dad and uncle, then hovered around the kitchen talking to Mum, Aunty Mal and Sajith until I thought I would burst.

I resisted the urge to use physical force to get him moving, and waited until he caught up with every member of my extended family before hurrying him out the door. The fresh air of the cool night smelt like freedom.

'Let's go mate!' I said, laughing.

Chan had chosen a movie – one of the *Pirates of the Caribbean* series. A movie night with a mate was just what the doctor ordered. Nothing too strenuous, just being out and about. As we walked into the theatre, I was suddenly conscious of what I looked like. My scalp was still blackened and the skin on my face peeled constantly. Half my face looked like a big red blister. I had worn long sleeves because it was cold and they covered up most of my bandaged arm. I was sticking to my chicks-dig-scars bravado mantra and I didn't want to move from that to being like Freddy from *Nightmare on Elm Street*.

I used jokes and quips to mask the little bit of reality that had crept unnoticed into my thoughts. I was still holidaying on the Island of Suppression.

People try not to be obvious when they stare at someone who is different, but that night I learnt – the hard way – that people look even more obvious when they are trying to not be obvious. There were lots of side glances and quickly repeated glances, downward glances that flicked up and then down again really quickly, double-take glances and pretending-to-suck-on-the-straw-and-drink-but-really-be-glancing glance. The most honest response was from a chubby five-year-old boy clutching a box of popcorn. There was no glancing there. He just stopped in the middle of the movie foyer, mouth agape, staring at me.

'G'day mate,' I said to the kid who ran scared, straight into the comforting arms of his nearby mother.

The short walk through the foyer was much harder than I had expected. When we look at people with disfigurements or disabilities, we never think that while we are watching them, they are watching *us* watching *them*. They notice.

'I think I just made that kid pee his pants,' I murmured to Chan.

'Are you sure it'd only be pee?' said Chan, smirking.

We both laughed as we walked into the darkened cinema. The dark proved an unexpected refuge. No one could see me. Everyone was the same. No one has a scarred face in the dark.

The movie was like the others in its franchise – lots of battles, swordfights and damsel saving. I was enjoying the movie until one scene made me catch my breath in horror. Johnny Depp's character, Jack Sparrow, was captured and hog-tied to a spit. A fire was ignited underneath him and the flames caught on his trousers. Depp kicked and blew on the fire and the audience laughed at the slapstick. But I didn't laugh – my reaction was to immediately break out in a cold sweat and start trembling. My breathing quickened and I sat frozen as the scene made me flash back to that night on the couch and my own fire.

Chan didn't notice and laughed along with the rest of the audience. By the time the film was finished, my reactions had calmed and I told Chan what had happened.

'Really?' he asked, clearly not even connecting that a scene in a film when someone is set on fire might be traumatic to someone who was actually recently set on fire.

I didn't discuss it at length, but instead, I analysed my response to the fire scene. I realised that it was probably normal for someone in my position to react as I had done. It also reminded me of something that we do with our patients. If a guy has done his back lifting a box, we ask him to lift a box as part of his therapy. Over and over I had seen really high levels of anxiety when I had asked people to do the thing that hurt them.

Now I understood – really understood – what I was asking them to do. Just like my reaction to the scene in the film, my patients were *scared* of what had hurt them, even if it was only a simple box.

Instead of going straight home – Chan and I went to a pub down the road from the movies. Being a weeknight, the pub was fairly empty and the few who were there looked like they'd been there for a while. A combination of dim lights and drunken patrons meant that I didn't get any stares. We spent an hour in a corner, enjoying a couple of quiet beers. I wasn't usually much of a drinker, but I could hold my own. On this night, my first drink since the attack, the beer went straight to my head.

'Anj, do you want to go home now?' Chan asked after a while.

'Nah, let's hang around a bit longer,' I said, even though my head was spinning with the two beers. The left side of my face felt as if a strong heat lamp was focused on it, and my arms felt like a thoroughfare for fire-ants. *Why was I in so much pain?* I was also really tired, and if Chan and I hadn't been talking, I would have nodded off. I felt like an old man: old, weary and in pain. But like any strapping 28-

year-old guy, I fought it. 'Let's get another drink... maybe a Coke.'

I fell asleep in the car on the way home. One minute I was chatting to Chan and my eyes were drooping. The next minute, Chan tapped my arm, saying we were home. I couldn't believe it. I'm a light sleeper and I've never dozed off on my way home, not even after a really big night. A movie, two beers and a Coke – was this all I could handle now? The logical part of my brain told me this was temporary. The wimpy-scared part of my brain wondered if this was who I was now.

I barely registered struggling into my pyjamas and crawling onto my mattress around midnight. I was aware of nothing until 1 pm the next day when I woke up with the sun on my face. I had slept thirteen hours straight, and boy, my whole body was aching!

The weird thing was that my mattress was on the floor of the lounge room and people had been coming in and out all morning, watching TV and chatting. Normally a light sleeper, I hadn't registered any of it.

How many times had I pointed out to my patients to avoid this overactivity–underactivity rollercoaster pattern? Halfway through the night, my body had told me that I was tired and in pain, but I was so desperate to do what I wanted to do, what I normally did, that I ignored it. Now I had to pay the price. It really was like being on a rollercoaster. I had overdone it, pushed myself beyond my limits, gone up in a rollercoaster, only to come crashing down. I felt stiff, sore and mentally drained – all this because of my relatively quiet night out with Chan.

I stumbled to the kitchen to get breakfast – more probably lunch at this time of day. What I had planned for the whole day was now out of whack. I would have to cancel my catch-up with my workmates that afternoon, to which I was really looking forward.

The only things I was going to get done today were my exercises and bandage change. The remainder of my day would be resting. Like an old man, a very cranky old man.

It was definitely a glimpse of life on the other side. I really understood why people push themselves – they want to resume living, they want to be who they were, they want to fight the change. It suddenly occurred to me that when I get better, I was going to be bloody good at my job because now I got it.

I understood.

PEELED LIKE A POTATO

For the next eight weeks, I had thrice-weekly appointments at the outpatients' clinic at Broomfield Hospital to get my dressings changed and have my progress monitored. Using my car, Dad drove me each time, without actually having a UK licence. Nothing was going to stop him from this duty to his son. I felt like a kid again as he made jokes about traffic jams and suburbs that had the same names as ones back home in Melbourne. Yes, I felt like a kid, a kid who'd heard all the same jokes a million times before. I wanted to laugh and shake my head but I held it in; I didn't want to encourage him.

Because I was a physiotherapist, my visits to the outpatients' clinic were mainly limited to dressing changes and wound cleaning. They didn't feel I needed physiotherapy because I already knew what I had to do. On one visit during my first week, the doctor inspected my arms and pointed to a large deeper burnt area on my left bicep muscle.

'You're going to need a skin graft on that,' he said.

'Can I do some abseiling before I get the skin graft?' I asked. I had raised money for ages for my work's staff abseiling charity fundraiser. I was going to get heaps of money for the local children's hospital. Some of my grip was returning and the thought of putting on some padded gloves, harnessing up and abseiling off the tower of the hospital where I worked and sailing down to the ground was so incredibly appealing at this particular moment.

Mum, who had come with me on this particular visit, slapped the back of my head. 'I don't think so!' she exclaimed, before the doctor even had a chance to reply.

'I guess if you want to...' said the doctor, 'we could postpone the skin graft.'

'No he is going to have his skin graft,' declared my mother. She turned to me, 'We came all this way to look after you – not for you to go jumping off buildings. Why are you trying to put us through more stress?'

'Okay, okay,' I said glumly, and turned to the doctor. 'I guess I won't be doing it.' The glimpse of freedom faded before my eyes. I would have to hand it over for someone else to do. Now that I wasn't going abseiling, the skin graft was scheduled for the following week.

My knowledge of skin grafts was minimal at best. I knew that they took skin from one part of your body and put it on another part of your body. Skin grafts had been a regular topic of conversation while I was in the burns unit.

When the doctor said that I needed one I agreed, of course, but inwardly, I was shaking my head. By this stage, I was sick of going in and out of hospital, sick of the smell, sick of the dim lighting, sick of the slow lifts, sick of the whole bloody lot. And now more.

None of my inner-rant could be repeated in front of Mum because she would feel sorry for herself and me and it just wouldn't help. This was a pattern that I was beginning to become really aware of – I had to hold my tongue about how I was feeling emotionally in order to protect the people who I loved and to guard them from any more distress. They were all doing so much to help – Mum and Dad had flown thousands of miles – it seemed churlish to whinge. I was also beginning to see that it was okay to talk about physical suffering, as long as you kept your emotional suffering to yourself.

I let out a sigh and added this new insight to the file in my brain that I would use for my patients when all of this was over. It occurred to me that all the pain patients over the last year that I had seen were doing the same thing; they often said that they didn't talk about their pain much at home because it distressed their families. When I asked how this made them *feel*, a common response was: *What do you mean, how do I feel? I'm in pain.* Now I understood that they couldn't separate the physical with the emotional aspects of pain. I, on the other hand, could separate them, but I couldn't talk about them. Maybe it was equally as damaging.

A week later, I arrived for an overnight stay at the hospital for my skin graft. I was given my own room for the first time in all of this. The surgeon looked me over and decided to take the skin for the graft from my right thigh. He explained that they would peel off a layer of skin – sort of like peeling a potato – and then place it over the most severely burnt part of my arm, the area over my left bicep muscle. Then they would stitch it on like a patch on a quilt.

I was knocked out for the actual procedure, but I felt it when I woke up again. Under a massive bandage on my leg, the graft site stung like a really bad graze, which, in fact, is what it was. I had gotten used to all my sore parts – arms, hands, face, and head. Now I had a new sore part – my thigh – and I was unreasonably frustrated by it.

During my studies, I learnt that there is a pain pathway that sends information from the injured site via the spinal cord to the brain. In the spinal cord part of the pathway, there are points – I imagined them to be like traffic lights on a highway – which turn green to let pain messages through. These lights are controlled not just by the pain messages but also the mood we are in. If we are in a good mood, we release endorphins that help turn the traffic lights to red, blocking pain messages and diminishing the pain we feel. If we are in a bad mood, angry or frustrated, we don't release endorphins and the traffic lights remain green, allowing through a barrage of pain messages for the brain to process. The way I was feeling, I reckoned that the traffic lights on my pain highway were stuck on green.

Once I realised that I felt such a strong sense of resentment towards this new pain, I used all my strength to try and switch my thinking around. *This is only short-term*, I told myself soothingly. *If you got through the burns, this is nothing. This is a minor set-back. Everything will be fine.* I slowed my breathing to try to get those lights to turn red again. Surprisingly, as soon as I calmed myself down, the pain lessened a bit. For now.

Despite my best and most reasoned efforts, my frustration built up again, like the rising waters in a boiling pan. I didn't notice it until I pulled back the sheets and tried to sit up. I wanted to get out of bed.

My mum jumped out of her chair and rushed over to guide my feet off the bed. 'Let me try and help you with your legs.'

'Just let it be!' I snapped. A shocked silence followed. I had never spoken disrespectfully to either of my parents. 'Sorry, I didn't mean to snap,' I gasped. *Deep breath. Calm down. It's not her fault; she's only trying to help.*

Mum looked uncertain and took a step back. Dad said nothing, and I realised suddenly that they were both silent because I was burnt. Any other time, Dad would have jumped to Mum's defence: *Don't talk to your mother like that!* But because I was burnt, all bets were off.

Not that I ever would, but I could see how easy it would be to turn mean in this situation. I had seen it plenty of times, but now I was *understanding* it profoundly for the first time. Someone in pain snaps at the people he or she loves who are trying to help. They don't say anything because the person is in pain. The person in pain snaps again with impunity. The family remain silent, and in the end, resentment seethes and bubbles beneath the surface and families can shatter. It was a nasty cycle that I would do anything to avoid.

'Um, can you help me to get my leg off the bed. Please.' It was a peace offering to Mum.

'Just do it slowly!' Mum's voice was caring and stern at the same time. The balance was restored.

I tried to move, but the pain in my thigh was almost unbearable. It stung like fire. And I'd had enough fire to last me a lifetime.

I hobbled over to the chair next to my bed and sat. It was good to be out of bed and I sat for almost two hours, eating the fruit and the biscuits that my parents had brought in for me. I sat while they fussed around, neatening my bed, picking up after me.

'What will we have to do for you at home?' asked Mum suddenly. She turned to Dad. 'How are we going to look after his leg? You will need to ask the doctor.'

'Will you calm down! They'll tell us!' Dad said with un-characteristic impatience.

I wasn't the only one on edge.

I sat like a child, watching this tiny war going on between my parents. Staring at my food, I pondered my situation and considered what lay ahead. For the first time, I realised that I may have to talk to someone about how I was feeling. As much as I wanted to avoid the emotional rollercoaster,

I had begun to realise that this wasn't about choosing to avoid it, but rather coping with its inevitable presence. But then again, maybe I just needed to cool off and everything would be fine again, I lied to myself.

But I didn't believe me.

I continued my outpatient sessions over the next six weeks. Every day, I spoke with Vin. Hearing her voice and talking to her made me feel stronger. To everyone around me, I was the patient, but to Vin thousands of kilometres away in Sydney, I was her new boyfriend, brave, upbeat, joking. I could hear the difference in my voice when I spoke to her. I might have been short with people around me and cranky, but as soon as that phone rang, I got the chance to be me. For her.

I told Vin about the people I met during my outpatient visits. At my appointments, I saw the same people come and go, all on their own healing journeys. Every time we got to the hospital door, there was a bloke in his mid thirties standing next to his motorbike smoking a cigarette. His son was the boy who had been burnt when his fishing rod had touched the electric wire causing burns to 95% of his body. I'd seen the father around the corridors. Every time Dad and I walked past his smoko, we always asked about his boy.

'My boy is strong,' he would say proudly, before telling me about whatever treatment his son was having that day.

'That's great,' I would say.

'I'm sure he'll get through this,' Dad would say with a confidence that made me cringe.

This tri-weekly exchange of hope and brightness was the game we all played. I was no expert, but I had never heard of anyone surviving burns to 95% of their body. Despite this, along with the devoted dad, my own father and I discussed the boy's new treatments with enthusiasm, and quietly hoped for a miracle.

For weeks, we saw the man and we spoke about his son and the numerous surgeries and skin grafts the boy had endured. Because he was always standing next to his motorbike, we discussed how great motorbikes were and how it felt to ride winding country roads. On the days we didn't see him, his motorcycle was there so we knew he was with his son. I felt for him, and so did Dad. I had seen how Dad had been the last time he had flown to my bedside after I suffered the collapsed lung. I remembered the look of helplessness in his eyes – and that was when I was recovering! Sometimes I wondered if it was actually harder on the parents watching their kids. It was one thing to feel the pain, but quite another to watch helplessly while someone you loved felt it.

Towards the conclusion of my outpatient appointments, there was no sign of the man or his motorcycle. The absence of the bike was eerie, and it stopped Dad and me in our tracks. It was most likely that the boy had lost his fight for life. I felt an immense wave of loss and sorrow, which I tried to push back by hoping with all my heart that the man wasn't there because his son had been transferred to another hospital.

There, but for the grace of God…

A NEW HOME

Staying at my uncle's house, surrounded by the intense love of Mum and Dad, I very quickly came to feel like a rare species in a zoo. It was like they needed to protect me and wrap me in cotton wool. I knew all of this came out of love, but it didn't stop me from feeling like I was going crazy.

Despite the renovations that had removed any traces of the fire-bomb attack, I just couldn't go back to the Bow house. Daily phone calls to Jill and Anita reinforced that they didn't want to be there either. The girls and I started looking through Gumtree – probably the most-used website in the UK for travellers wanting accommodation. One day, we struck gold.

I held the phone clumsily in my newly-unwrapped hands. It had been seven weeks since the attack, and while my arms were red-raw, tiny bits of pigment on my hands were starting to become visible, which meant that I was healing.

'Anj!' said Jill with excitement. 'I think we found a place! It's in Leytonstone. It has three bedrooms. Looks perfect. The kitchen...' She talked at a million miles an hour.

I couldn't keep up. 'Hold on,' I laughed. 'Where is it again? How much are they asking?'

'Leytonstone. Anita and I want to see it. Can you come too?'

An opportunity to get out and about was too good to decline. I had left my uncle's house for my trips to the hospital and a couple of trips out with Chan, and that was it.

A few days later, I got into my car and drove to pick up the girls. Being able to drive again gave me feelings of freedom that made me want to shout from the rooftops: *I am free at last!*

Mum and Dad stood in the driveway, waving goodbye and shouting instructions as I got into the car.

Dad: *Drive carefully. Don't speed. Don't stay out too long. You need your rest.*

Mum: *Call us when you get there. Don't eat junk food; I'll cook you something healthy when you get home.*

I shut the door on their advice, smiling to reassure them. I loved them and wanted to escape from them in equal measures.

When you get burnt, for ages afterwards, everything you touch feels hot. My nerve endings were growing back and repairing themselves but they were sensitive to everything. My need to get out of the house and regain my independence meant that I had to ignore the pain as much as I could. The nearest thing I could compare driving to, with my new ultra-sensitive nerve endings, was getting into your car on a really hot day after it's been parked in the sun. You flick the gear stick really fast and try not to touch the steering wheel any more than you have to. I found myself driving with the loosest grip I could manage.

But at least I was driving.

I made it to the Bow house and parked right out the front. My energy had been so focused on driving and trying to minimise the burning sensations in my raw hands, that I didn't really give much thought to returning to the house.

I used my key and felt the new slowness of my actions. It was like I was battery operated and my batteries were running flat. My frustration was tempered by the huge relief that at least I could use my hands to get the key into the lock. I knew lots of people through my work who couldn't even do that. The clinician in me also knew that these things take time.

When the girls came bounding down the stairs to greet me, I felt a sense of renewal. They both hugged me, but I couldn't hug them back yet because of my arms. Nonetheless, this was just like old times.

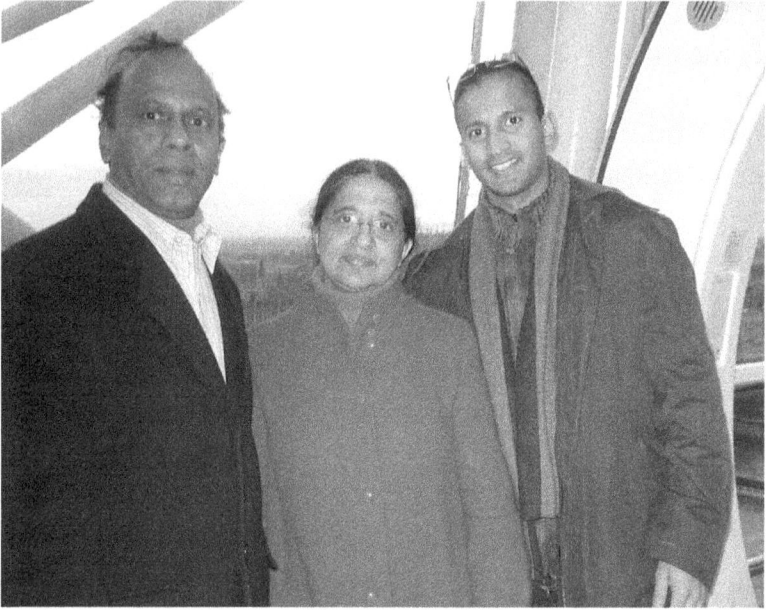

On the London Eye with my parents

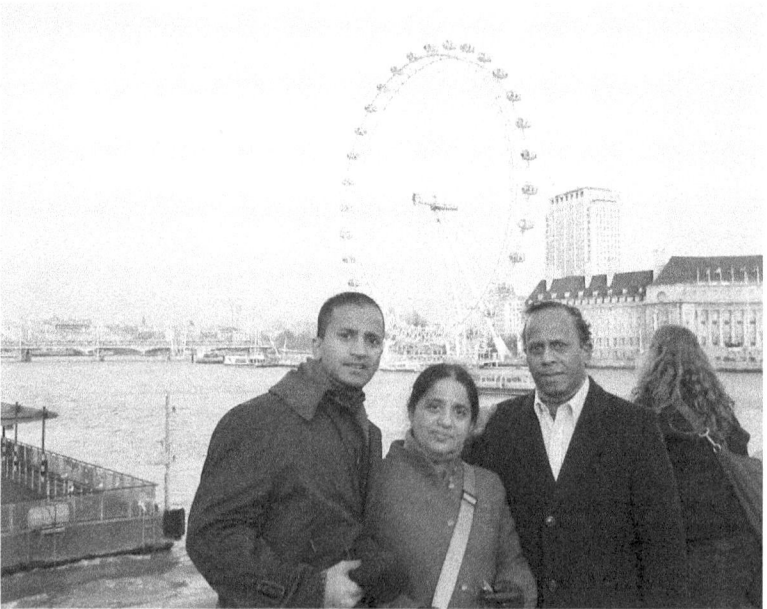

A sunny, yet wintry day on Westminster Bridge

The house in Leytonstone was only a couple of suburbs further out than Bow. Without saying anything to the girls, I looked around for council estates. I didn't want to get caught in the middle of any more incidents of gang warfare – if that's what it was that caused my attack. After the visit from the earnest cop when I was in hospital, I hadn't heard back from the police.

The house in Leytonstone was old with creaky floor boards. It was on a quiet street with no council estates in sight. The train station and the local pub were a short walk away, and there was a convenience store a few doors down. It was perfect. The house had high ceilings and all the bedrooms were upstairs. The front bedroom was the biggest by far.

'Can I have this one?' I asked. The studies for my Master's degree were due to begin in a couple of weeks and I would need study space as well. 'This is perfect. I can put my desk here, my bed here, my books here…' In minutes, I had mentally placed all my furniture in this new big room. The front window overlooked the street. I definitely wasn't going to put my bed there, but I could put my study desk there where there was plenty of natural light for when I hit the books. I would put my bed away from the window, just so I could close my eyes in peace.

The downstairs lounge was huge but it smelt a bit damp. In one corner was an old piano. The kitchen was also large and it even had a cellar, dimly illuminated by a single light bulb dangling from a wire. I carefully walked down the narrow creaky wooden staircase. It was damp down there and filled with wooden planks, dirt, old mattresses and cardboard boxes.

Aside from the junk-filled cellar, the rest of the house was great and much bigger than the Bow house. We all loved it.

Within a week, we found ourselves in the real estate office signing the contract. The estate agent who was doing the paperwork for us was a guy in his mid-thirties. We had been shown into his office and he stood from behind his desk and shook hands with the girls. I held back because I wasn't up to shaking hands yet. We all sat down and he shuffled through the papers we needed to sign.

Every now and then, he would glance at my arms. I had my sleeves rolled up because it was a hot day. His glances were obvious to both me and the girls. I chose to ignore it; Jill didn't.

'He was hit with a petrol bomb,' she said, forthrightly. 'But it wasn't his fault; it was a case of mistaken identity.'

'Um... okay,' said the estate agent, quickly looking down at his papers. 'Did they catch them?'

'No. The police are still looking for them,' said Jill.

'Hope they catch them,' said the agent awkwardly.

It suddenly struck me that I hadn't given much thought to the two bombers being caught. I guess that I had a couple of moments when I fantasised about them being caught and me dousing them with petrol and standing over them with a flame – just so that they could know what I felt like, and to understand the horror of their actions. But aside from that, I realised that it made no difference to me if they were caught. My wounds wouldn't suddenly be healed if they were caught. Nothing would change. I also knew that to be festering with anger and resentment was not good for my healing. As much as I could muster, my mind had to remain switched to positive.

I went home that day and shared our excitement with my parents who, true to form, mixed their happiness for me with their worries about me, and expressed both in equal measure. As soon as I gave them our moving date, my dad was on the phone trying to track down one of his friends to see if he could help out. Even on the other side of the world, Dad could find a friend to call in a favour. It was a typical Sri Lankan trait – whenever you meet someone for the first time, you always try to make some sort of connection. When Sri Lankans meet each other, it's like a game of extreme six-degrees of separation takes place. The first thing Sri Lankans do is work out how they know each other, how they might be related or which friends they might have in common. Once these connections are made, they are made for life. Once, I had to help out my mum's sister's husband's brother-in-law's daughter from Perth who wanted to find somewhere to live in Melbourne.

As expected, Dad found a long lost friend who offered his courier van to move our stuff. Mum and Dad helped with the move and loved the house as soon as they saw it. Their approval was weirdly comforting; if I got their approval, maybe it would be a safe place.

After a long day of moving, we all gathered around exhausted. It really took it out of me. My back was sore and my arms were throbbing, yet I had hardly done anything. My folks planned to stay the night and Jill started dinner.

'Anj!' Jill called from the kitchen. 'How the hell do you work the oven? I can't see the flame.'

'Hold on,' I yelled from upstairs. 'I'll come and take a look at it.' It was a nice feeling showing my folks that I was the man of the house. It was a nice switch from being the patient of the house. They followed me downstairs. No doubt, Mum would insist on helping with the cooking.

'What's the matter? Let me have a look,' I said, squatting down to peer into the old oven.

'It won't light,' said Jill.

I pressed the ignition switch and turned the gas valve on. There was an immediate *hiss* of gas. 'Hmmm... the gas is working but the ignition switch isn't.' I would have to light the oven manually. We didn't have one of those hand-held long-nosed igniters – instead I rolled-up some old news paper and lit one end.

I tried to reach into the oven. The *hiss* of gas was louder than it should be, magnified by a sudden feeling in my very core.

Thump, thump.

My heart pounded hard.

Thump, thump.

My arm trembled as if it was possessed.

Thump, thump.

I just couldn't force my arm to go inside.

Thump, thump.

Gees Anj, get a grip, I told myself. *Just do it. If anything happens, you go to the hospital. They'll fix you. At least this time, you'll be ready for whatever.*

I pushed my shaking scarred arm deep into the dark hissing oven to light the burner.

What was all that about?

'Ha! Talk about shaky old-man hands,' I joked.

Everyone laughed out of courtesy. Then the moment was gone.

MY SYDNEY LIFELINE

If I wasn't being honest to the people around me about how I was really feeling, I did at least have one life-line: Vin in Sydney. We were in daily contact, either by long phone conversations or short text messages.

'I tried to light the oven today and I was shitting myself,' I told her. 'I couldn't believe it.'

'What do you mean?' she asked from her desk in Sydney. Her day was my night.

'I tried to light the oven with a bit of rolled up newspaper and I panicked.'

Vin laughed. 'No wonder! You've just been burnt! I would be scared too if I had been burnt and I had to light an old oven with a naked flame.'

Of course.

Even from the other side of the world, Vin managed to be my lifeline, my voice of reason. I could bounce things off her without worrying that she would take any action or stop me from doing anything or tell my parents and make them worry even more. She was *safe*!

I settled into my new life like an engine on idle. I was really fortunate that my work was paying me sick-pay and money wasn't a problem. On a typical day, I would wake up feeling exhausted, say goodbye to the girls as they left for work, kill time during the morning pacing up and down the house and watching useless TV, do my boring 'Twinkle Twinkle Little 'Star' finger exercises, have something to eat for lunch, go for a walk around the block, ponder why all this happened to me, and then call some friends and leave messages on answering machines.

I spent hours during the day lying in bed, dozing off and waking. Of course, the consequence of sleeping through much of the day meant being wide awake most nights, until the small – and lonely – hours of the morning. Some nights, I would talk on the phone to Vin, but most nights, I just twiddled my sore thumbs. It didn't take long for me to not even know what time or what day it was. My body clock was spinning out of control and I couldn't seem to do anything about it. The only exciting part of the day was when the girls returned home after work.

I was like a sponge, wanting to know every detail about their lives on the *outside*. We would sit around, chatting and laughing, and for the hours between them getting home and them going to bed, I felt alive and normal. Then the long lonely night stretched out before me, leaving me alone and isolated from the world.

To everybody around me, I looked like I was recovering, getting back to the old me. But it was a façade. There were two Anjelos – one was the funny guy who could keep laughing despite his new scars. The other was a lonely isolated fearful young man who had lost his place and purpose in the world.

Two weeks after I moved into my new house, my parents returned to Melbourne. It was my cue to get back into a routine, but *what* routine?

While I was able to use Vin as a lifeline for some stuff, I was very conscious of not coming across as a whinger to my new girlfriend. I knew that my salvation, no matter what support networks I had, was ultimately up to me.

It really was time to use what I knew through my work as a pain management specialist and start applying it to myself.

It was another case of practising what I preached.

GUITAR HERO

The thing I preached most to my patients was the importance of having a structured routine. Being physically and mentally active during the day meant that at night, the mind and body would be fatigued and able to rest. Not having a structured routine meant that my body was not fatigued enough to sleep well and I was becoming lethargic. It dawned on me that I was living the very life I tried to help change for my patients.

Around three months after the attack, my pain was still persisting, putting it in the chronic pain category. I already knew what it was like to have chronic pain. I still had back pain from the surgery for my collapsed lung nearly a year earlier.

But this was not just pain; I was also experiencing really weird sensations. If I was in the sun, the left side of my face would feel as if a hot ray lamp was on it. My arms regularly had tingling low-current electric shocks running through them. I also hadn't regained much dexterity in my fingers, which were still rough and sore. My frustration levels were also higher because, even though I wanted to get back to work, I couldn't because the risk of infection was too great from my burns that had not completely healed. If I scratched at my arms, which itched a lot, I risked breaking the skin of some of the tiny blisters that still covered the burn-sites. Even using super-human efforts not to scratch, sometimes I just couldn't help it.

One day, I called the hospital and spoke to a doctor. 'My hands are still sore, and I still have the pain in the arms,' I said, frustrated.

'You just have to rest and take it easy. Go see your GP and get some stronger medication,' the doctor suggested.

'Thanks anyway,' I said, putting down the receiver.

Resting and taking it easy wasn't helping. Rest and take pills: that seemed to be the standard response. I should have guessed and saved myself the phone call. How often had I listened to chronic pain patients telling me that their own doctors said the same thing? Rest and pills. If only it was that easy.

Not only didn't the rest-and-pills mantra help, it was actually counter-productive. After an injury, moderate activity in between short rest breaks is vital. It keeps the body healthy and the brain distracted from the pain.

I figured that I would need to take charge of my own re-habilitation and make it a bit more interesting. The key to a good rehabilitation is to find physical activities that you enjoy doing. I started by changing my hospital-sanctioned exercises; finger wriggling just wasn't doing it for me. I always recommended to my patients that they should find something that they enjoy because they are more likely to stick with it. Let's face it, if you don't enjoy general exercise programs, you're not likely to continue them into the future.

It was then that I noticed my guitar leaning against my work desk and had an idea. I got my guitar-for-beginners book out and thumbed through it. The book taught the enthusiast how to play songs using just three chords: C, F and G. Most were Beatles' songs. Finally, an enjoyable way to do my exercises, something I could put my mind to. It was another light-bulb moment for me as a clinician. I needed to make sure that my patients' exercise programs were interesting and meaningful to them, or at least a stepping stone towards a more enjoyable activity.

So I began to teach myself the guitar, chord by chord. It was painful to hold the neck of the guitar and press my sensitive fingertips into the metal strings to change chords, but I did what I could manage.

Before long, it was music to my ears, awkward and discordant music, but music nonetheless.

One afternoon, in the empty house, I felt ready. I belted out my first complete Beatles tune, strumming my guitar and singing at the top of my lungs.

My fingertips felt as if they were under a red-hot heater, but my smile from ear to ear said it all.

THE THREE BASIC INGREDIENTS OF A GOOD LIFE

Guitar practice continued but soon I craved more interesting things to do. Those three basic ingredients to a good life became all the more relevant: someone to love, something to do and something to look forward to. If you have all three, you are in a pretty good place.

I had someone to love, but I needed more to do, and I definitely craved something to look forward to. As if the gods heard me, one day, Vicky, my boss, called.

'Anjelo, how are you?' she asked in concerned voice.

'I'm okay, but staying home is doing my head in,' I told her.

There was a pause in the conversation. Then Vicky said, 'Well, I'm sure we can find something for you to do from home, if you like.'

'Anything! I'll do it. Just email me.' The excitement in my voice surprised me. I was clearly desperate. We spoke for about twenty minutes. I updated her on my recovery and laughed about my guitar efforts. She told me what was going on at work, which was surprisingly interesting. It really made me appreciate what we said to clients all the time: work isn't just work, it's also a social network. Friday night drinks, gossip sessions, lunchtime jogging, hearing about what people got up to on the weekend, planning the next staff social event. I drank in the inconsequential details like a Jack Daniel's at a bar.

Within five minutes of me hanging up the receiver, I had mail in my inbox. Vicky had forwarded me some research articles to summarise. For the first time in weeks, I felt as if I had *something to do* that was really worthwhile. I was useful again.

Work is crucial to our lives. It makes us feel like we are contributing to something bigger. It makes us feel valued. Through work, we achieve things. Work is often the last thing on the minds of people who are injured. I knew it was vital to get back to work as soon as I possibly could. If the summarising task could make me feel excited and purposeful, imagine what really going back to work could do for me.

Vicky had sent through half a dozen articles and I decided to pace myself through them, even though a part of me wanted to sit up all night and get them all done. I was fully aware that my concentration span had suffered a major blow through all of this. I figured one article a day would be manageable.

I immediately started reading the first article. I took regular breaks to stretch and walk around the house. I made sure I was comfortable. Now that I had something to do, I wanted to be the textbook example of recovery. Finally.

The second article on the second day was easier and my concentration definitely improved. The third day was even better. I was elated. I was purposeful. I finished all six articles in six days and emailed my summaries back to Vicky. I followed the email with a phone call asking for more work.

Now that I was on a better and more purposeful road to recovery, I started to think of the future. What were my goals? I teach my patients the importance of goals and now it was my turn.

After some thought, I decided that my goal could be

to get back to work within the next four weeks. A second goal was that I wanted to be fully fit to begin studying for my Master's degree, which would begin in around six weeks. And while I was at it, I made another goal to run around the neighbourhood in two weeks. My fitness was important. I still hadn't given up the thought of finishing my London adventure by going home via the Himalayas. But the trek to the Everest base camp would require a level of fitness that I no longer possessed and needed to get back. The thought of achieving my childhood dream gave me a tangible third ingredient: *something to look forward to*.

For two weeks, everything was working well. I started running. I typed for longer. I rode my motorbike again. Even my guitar playing sounded better. I swear. My nightly conversations or texts with Vin were upbeat. Of course, the pain and some of those weird symptoms persisted, some days more than others, but it felt as if I was finally getting on with my life.

Every day, I could see the light at the end of the tunnel getting brighter and brighter.

Unfortunately for me, the light at the end of the tunnel turned out to be an oncoming train.

THE ONCOMING TRAIN

It started as just another weekday. A good friend from Melbourne was in London and staying with her friend close by. I donned my leathers and shot off to meet with her for lunch. I was free as a bird riding my bike. Until now, I had ridden it locally and gradually adjusted to the different sensations of tightness as I gripped the handles with my slowly-healing hands.

We had lunch at a local pub and I downed a large pint of Coke. After lunch, I excused myself to go to the toilet. It had been a very long time since I had donned my leathers, and it was a struggle to unzip my pants with sensitive fingers.

With the relief of finally getting my fly undone and being able to pee, came an uncomfortable, burning sensation in the waterworks when I had finished. *This was odd.* The burning sensation lingered, and when I got back inside, I ordered a pint of water. *Maybe water might sort it out,* I thought to myself.

As I was riding back home, I had the urge to pee again. An urgent urge. I hurriedly pulled into a McDonald's and ran into the toilet. I peed but at the end of it was agony. I felt as if I had peed boiling water or razor blades. More alarming than the pain were the droplets of blood-stained urine.

What was happening? Panic hit. I struggled to hold back tears. I couldn't take anything else going wrong. I just couldn't.

I rode home as quickly as I could and I soon had to pee again. This time there were only trickles of urine but there was more blood. Why was this happening to me? All I wanted was to move on with my life, to get better. Anger, helplessness and self-pity draped me like a shroud. I was making my way downstairs, trying to figure out my next move just as Anita came home.

'Anita, I need to go to the hospital again. I'm peeing blood,' I told her in a panicked voice.

'What?' she said, shocked.

'I don't know what's going on. Can you take me to the hospital?'

In the Accident and Emergency department of the local hospital, I described my symptoms to the doctor.

'Looks like you have a UTI,' he said.

'Urinary tract infection? How?' It didn't make sense but then again, lately, nothing with my body seemed to make sense.

Do you have protected sex? How many sexual partners do you have? Do you have unprotected anal sex?' The doctor, of Bangladeshi origin, asked his list of mandatory questions.

What drug is this guy on?

'Mate, I've been in and out of the hospital for the past four months. I haven't had time for any sex; besides, my girlfriend lives in Sydney.'

'It could be because of the dehydration following your burns, or the strong medications you were on,' the doctor said, having ruled out a sexual cause. 'Your kidneys need to keep filtering fluid, and the amount of fluid is affected after serious burns.'

Over the next two weeks, I tried different antibiotics and was in and out of hospital because the infection wasn't resolving. I was eventually referred to a specialist who prescribed an antibiotic that worked.

Nonetheless, the UTI was the straw that broke the camel's back. My emotions were spiralling out of control. I just couldn't control myself. I was angry, frustrated and helpless, completely at the whim of my traitorous body. I slept curled up like a lonely child, and most nights, cried myself to sleep.

I wasn't coping. I couldn't take this anymore. How many times would I have to fight to be well? How many battles did I have left?

Completely withdrawn, I couldn't even bring myself to consider socialising, even with the girls at home. Over the sleepless, pain-filled nights, one thought pulsated in my mind. I wanted to go back to Melbourne, to go home. Home was a beacon. Home was safe.

I didn't tell the girls how I was feeling. I didn't want to leave them *alone* again, and I didn't want to give up on my Master's degree. My mind was like a washing machine, churning this way and that.

Something else started to concern me. I became increasingly fearful of walking outside. What else might happen? My run of bad luck made anything seem possible. I couldn't help but look over my shoulder as I walked down the street. If I was having a conversation with a friend, my eyes would dart around the room for possible threats. When one friend pointed this out to me, I was surprised. I didn't know I was doing it.

I wanted a tattoo on my forehead saying: *I am Australian. I mean no harm to anyone.* And then, perhaps, harm would leave me alone too.

During a telephone call to Vin, she could hear my despair.

'Come home,' she said.

We had planned for her to come over and work in the UK so that we could be together while I completed my Master's degree.

'But our plans...' my voice trailed off.

'Anj, you're not happy there any more. There's no point forcing yourself to stay. We can do London together another time. You need to get yourself better first.

'But what about Everest base camp?' I felt so hopeless. Just when my dream was almost within reach, I knew I just couldn't do it. My heart was no longer in it. The pull of home was greater than my boyhood dream.

'Anj, the Everest base camp isn't going anywhere.'

She spent hours talking me into going home, and I spent hours being persuaded by her arguments. Before long, she was preaching to the choir.

Finally, I started back at work again. My boss had been wonderful and had done her best to accommodate me. It was great to be back among friends, but even they started telling me I needed to go back to Melbourne. Maybe they could see it in my eyes.

While work brought some blessed relief, the problem was going home afterwards. I dreaded the thought of sleeping alone, curled up with my thoughts. The girls did their best but I just couldn't get myself out of whatever it was that I was in – a very dark place.

On the day I made the decision to leave, I told Jill and Anita, expecting they would understand and be sympathetic. I was wrong.

It felt like my two precious friends had turned on me like vipers. Well, it wasn't that bad; just my perception really. But, that's what tends to happen when you're traumatised:

irrational thinking, emotions become amplified, and perception becomes reality. The girls were just venting their frustration, not turning into deadly snakes.

'How can you just leave us?' exclaimed Anita. 'We moved here so we could all be together!'

'I just can't do it anymore,' I implored. 'It's all too hard.'

'What do you mean?' huffed Jill. 'It was just a urinary tract infection! Girls get them all the time.'

'It's not just that; it's everything,' I said with tears in my eyes. Any fight I had left in me had gone a long time ago.

'But we went through it too,' said Anita indignantly. 'Just when we're all back to normal, you're going to ruin it.'

I suddenly felt angry and betrayed. How could they not understand that I needed to go? The people at work were all telling me to go home. How could my closest friends not see it too? It took me some time before I finally understood.

After such closeness, my final weeks with the girls were frosty. I helped them find a replacement housemate – a male kick-boxer from New Zealand. He was the best applicant given the circumstances. They would be in safe hands.

The day I left, there was no send off. The girls left for work without as much as a goodbye. I left a bottle of wine on the kitchen table with a thank-you card:

> *Thank you for being there for me. I will never forget all the help you gave me during my difficult times.*
> *Love Anj*

I wheeled my suitcase to my car that was already loaded with the rest of my stuff. After I closed the boot on the suitcase, I climbed into the driver's seat and looked towards the house. I took a couple of deep breaths then slowly nodded my head. Yes, I was good to go.

I spent my final three weeks in the UK in Kent with Uncle Jine, Aunt Mal and my cousins. It was the three weeks leading up to Christmas when the pain clinic closes for the holidays. I had arranged to spend Christmas with my aunt and uncle, and then leave before the New Year. In my spare moments, I pondered the reasons why Jill and Anita had turned on me. It just didn't make any sense. Can love turn to hate so quickly? Had I just imagined our closeness? A small part of me was frustrated that they couldn't see why I had to go.

When these thoughts refused to stop swirling around in my head, I realised that it was time to seek help; it could no longer wait. First the collapsed lung, then the turmoil of surgery, then getting hit with a petrol bomb when I thought I was getting back on track, then while recovering from that, having the painful urinary tract infection and then the situation with the girls. It was too much for me to deal with on my own.

I booked myself an appointment with the staff counsellor at my work. I always promoted the importance of counselling in my teaching, but I never thought that I would need it. It was difficult walking into my first session.

As much as I advocated counselling, it felt as if it was weak of me, a therapist myself, to need therapy. Quickly, I challenged this. *I am only human; not only do I need to deal with someone trying to kill me, but I also need to deal with my collapsed lung, just eight months earlier. It is only natural that I need help. Just like someone may need my help to sort out their sore back, I need the help of a counsellor to sort out my emotions.*

Sitting opposite her in a session, I was able to open up to her like I hadn't to anyone else. I told her about everything: the attack, the slow healing, the frustrations, the house move, and finally, how the girls had reacted to my decision to leave.

After much discussion, I began to understand why the girls reacted like they had. They had been through a horrific event, but unlike me, they didn't have the benefit of the support that I did. While I was lying in hospital surrounded by friends and family and treatment and support, the girls had to live in the bombed house, a house in which they had seen their dear friend nearly killed. Not only this but, they had lived at the back of the house for weeks, mainly in the kitchen and the back bedroom, because they feared for their lives. To add to this, none of their friends had recognised the extent of the girls' emotional scars either, assuming that they were okay simply because the Molotov cocktail had hit me, not them.

And when things almost got back to normal, after visiting me in hospital, after looking after me on the first night out of hospital, and after we had just moved to a new house, I decide to leave. It must have felt like the group that they had fought so hard to keep together was breaking up, on my call, just like Anita had said. They too were victims of the attack, and I had failed to appreciate the true extent of this.

The counsellor helped me to more fully understand what we had all been through and what it meant now. After a handful of sessions with her, I felt lighter. After the fire-bomb attack, I had so much to do just to get through each day. I was so focused on physical healing, that I probably ignored the emotional healing. This experience made me see that both types of healing have equal importance. You can't separate the body from the soul.

For the first time, I felt like my future did contain a light at the end of the tunnel. A real light this time, not a train. My aunt, uncle and cousins all came to the airport to see me off. I had taken them on such a rollercoaster during my stay there, but they stuck by me above and beyond the call of family duty.

It was hard saying goodbye, but I got on the flight with a clear focus for a fresh start. As the sound of the jet engine roared, I leaned back into the seat and hoped against hope that I had made the right choice.

I watched out the window as England slipped away and was replaced by grey wintry clouds. When we broke through, I saw an expanse of clear blue skies ahead.

COMING HOME

I landed in Melbourne just in time to see in the New Year of 2007. I was welcomed into the arms of my own family at Tullamarine Airport. When the plane's wheels had screeched down the tarmac, I didn't get the overwhelming sense of home that I'd imagined. It had been four years since I had lived in Melbourne, four years since I'd had a life here.

Mum was smack-bang front-row-centre behind the rail as the automatic doors of customs opened. As she waved and smiled, I took in a deep breath and let it out. My mother's beaming face and possessive hug epitomised my ambivalence. I loved my family and they were so important to me, but I was returning home slightly worse for wear at twenty-eight years of age.

My mother's hug was joined by my father's, and I was surrounded by their love, a great big protective bubble of love.

My bedroom at home was exactly how I had left it, only cleaner. My absence hadn't stopped Dad vacuuming it every week as if I had never left home in the first place. Mum and Dad lived happily in this kind of denial. They would even ring me in the UK and ask permission if any of their friends were staying and they needed to use my room. Mum had re-washed every item of clothing I'd ever owned and it was all neatly folded ready for me to step back into my old life. Dad had ironed all my shirts and they were all lined up in my closet in neat rows.

My big upstairs bedroom was full of summer light, and it was safe. And even though it was at the front of the house, a big front yard put space between me and the footpath. Not that I even thought of that because petrol bombs don't happen in new housing estates in Wantirna.

On a full stomach of home-cooked curry, I lay down on my comfy bed to sleep off my jet-lag. It had been six months since the petrol bomb, and I returned to my big safe bedroom looking only a little different to when I had left. My forehead and the skin graft on my arm were still a little patchy, my ear had almost healed, and my left arm and hand had fading scars. The doctors in London had been amazed at how well I'd healed. I still experienced an intermittent unpleasant tingling in both arms, which hot weather could turn into a stinging itchy sensation. I knew I would have to be careful in the Aussie summer sun because the skin on my arms and head was only six-months old and would burn like a baby. My upper back regularly ached as a result of the collapsed lung surgery. Oddly, the pain was a mirror image of the scar site; the scar from the surgery was on the left, yet the pain was more on the right side. At its worst, it feels like someone is rubbing broken glass into my skin. If I used my hands a lot, they felt arthritic, making hands-on treatments for my patients quite difficult. My hands had become more sensitive to the Deep Heat-type creams that physios often used on patients.

Four years earlier, I walked out of my parents' house fit as a fiddle, and now I had returned with pains that persisted long enough to put them in the category of chronic pain. My injuries and their ongoing repercussions meant that I had to consider a different kind of work. Teaching self-management strategies to people in pain at the pain clinic in London had worked perfectly for me because we didn't do any hands-on treatment there. I would have to seek a similar job here, but my online research had shown that there weren't many of these around. Another option that I could consider was occupational rehabilitation and helping injured workers return to their jobs.

These thoughts wandered through my mind as the jet-lag won, and I drifted off to the best sleep I'd had in six months.

In the first couple of days home, every relative I'd ever met, and some I hadn't, came to visit my parents' prodigal son. The house wafted with the smells of all my favourite dishes: chicken biryani, prawn curry, calamari curry, Chinese rolls and chocolate cake.

'You need to put on more weight,' Mum kept saying as she put yet another plate of something delicious in front of me.

I lapped it up as I lived like a king over the long summer of 2007. Mum cooked and washed while Dad did all my ironing and cleaning. Friends visited. Life was sweet.

But there is always a small downside. The cost of all this king-living was that parents are always parents, especially Sri Lankan ones.

Not long after I returned, a bunch of my cousins organised a night out at a club. We had a great night catching up and dancing. My mobile phone rang at three in the morning, just as we were heading home. It was Dad.

'I'm just ringing to find out what time you're coming home,' he asked casually.

I was glad he couldn't see my eyes rolling. 'Dad, I'm twenty-nine!' I laughed.

'Okay,' he said apologetically, 'I'll go back to sleep.'

One thing that I did notice when I caught up with friends whom I hadn't seen for a couple of years, was that they all felt sorry for me.

'I can't believe that happened to you,' they would say. 'I'm so sorry this happened. You don't deserve this. If only the guys that did this had got the right house.'

No! That was so far away from my thinking. There was a mother and child in the 'right' house.

What people imagined for me was very different from the picture I saw of myself. I found myself trying to explain it to them. Good can come from bad. The things that had happened to me had made me different, humble even. The collapsed lung and the petrol bomb had changed me from the gung-ho guy I had been to someone who appreciates the things I have rather than focusing on the things I don't have. I was now someone who knew that a truth had come from these experiences. This was especially true in my work. I wasn't just a guy telling people in pain how to lead a better life; I was the guy who had swum the murky waters of pain and come out okay. Patients *listened* to me. We connected on a different level.

I *knew* and they knew I knew.

Another thing I gained was that I had been tested and I had passed the test. I knew that when I was put under the pump, I would come out okay. When I told the story of getting myself into the cold shower after the attack, people shook their heads in wonder and told me that they wouldn't have had the presence of mind to do that. The more I saw my story reflected in the incredulity of others, the more sure I became that I could handle anything.

That was why the expressions of sorrow were so alien. The picture others saw of me was very different to the picture I saw of myself.

Vin and I had been in almost daily email or phone

contact before the fire-bomb. Since I'd been home, knowing that she was only a one-hour plane trip away was hard. She wanted to let me settle in before she flew down to Melbourne.

On 12 January, Dad and I drove to Avalon Airport to pick her up. I waited nervously at the gate as Dad kept an eye on the arrivals screen.

Vin stepped off the plane and I quickly picked her out among the rest of the passengers as they spilt out of the luggage shed at Avalon airport: my 5 ft gremlin on steroids.

It was the first time I had laid eyes on her since she had become my girlfriend.

I grinned to myself as I watched her. It was like watching one of those TV shows where the camera crew is waiting for the reunion.

'Vin!' I called.

She saw me and smiled a smile that lit up her face. She hurried over and her eyes darted for a second from my face to my arms. Looking. Then we hugged.

'How are you? How was the flight?' I didn't know what else to say. I was so good at speaking for hours over the phone, but suddenly I had stage fright.

'Yeah good. How are you?' I think she felt the same.

'Good,' I said. It was fifty per cent good and fifty per cent awkward, mostly on account of Dad being there. A passionate embrace like you see in the movies was out of the question if your dad is looking on.

Vin loved meeting my family because she loved being the centre of attention. Dad fussed over her and carried her bags to the car. While my father was enthusiastic and welcoming, Mum was a little more reserved towards this woman who could potentially take her son away. Her questions were definitely the questions of a suspicious potential mother-in-law, worked into casual conversation. 'Can you cook?

Do you live with your parents? Do you want to live in Melbourne?'

Vin lived with her parents, helped her mother cook and loved Melbourne. In other words, she passed Mum's initial tests. Round one complete. Mum's questions about how many babies Vin wanted would have to wait till next time. Another thing that Mum approved of was that Vin was one of a twin. Mum loved twins.

Between Mum and Dad, and Vin meeting about forty members of my extended family during the course of her weekend stay, we didn't have a lot of time alone. This wasn't helped by Dad firmly putting Vin's suitcase in the spare bedroom and Mum leaving the guest towel set on the spare bed.

Any other sleeping arrangement was absolutely and unequivocally out of the question. And the question itself was never asked.

I loved the vibe that Vin gave off. She was energetic and positive and people around her rode the wave of her energy. We laughed and joked and in what felt like minutes, the weekend was over and I was putting her back on a plane with promises that I would come up and meet her family soon.

When I did meet Vin's family, her parents were polite and treated me as a mere friend of their daughter's. I wasn't from their caste of Gujarati and not only that, I wasn't even Indian. In those early meetings, I think Vin's parents lived happily in complete denial. In that way, they had a lot in common with my parents who used denial to great effect all the time. Vin's family didn't have a spare room, so I stayed at a motel down the road.

By the end of my visit to Sydney, we agreed to do the long-distance relationship until Vin made the decision to move to Melbourne. I was adamant that she needed to *want* to move for herself, not feel that she was forced to because of me. Vin planned to test the waters at the big accounting firm where she worked to see if a transfer to their Melbourne office was possible.

For now, it was a waiting game.

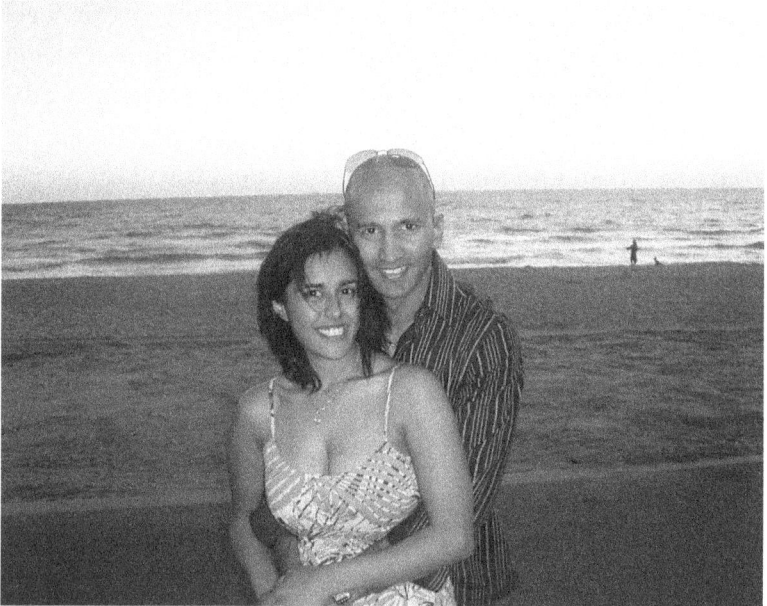

Vin and I at St Kilda Beach, Melbourne

BACK TO WORK

My summer of bumming around at home and getting stronger soon ended. I basked in being looked after and fussed over, but then it was time to start looking for work. In a lot of ways, it would have been easier to find a place of my own, but that was a mine-field in a Sri Lankan family. If Vin moved down from Sydney and I moved in with her, we would incur the wrath of both families, and any chance of inter-familial approval would be zero. Our relationship would have to occur in a banished wasteland, even in this day and age.

Things had to be done correctly along the tightrope of inter-cultural sensitivities. If Vin moved to Melbourne, she would get her own place.

By the end of January, I had set the feelers out to see what work would best suit me. A job came up with an occupational rehabilitation provider. The job was in Port Melbourne, over an hour's drive from Wantirna. Nonetheless, I wanted to remain with Mum and Dad, to save money and also to give them a chance to have me back home.

My job was to help people with injuries return to work. It didn't take me long to realise that there was a need for a quality chronic pain service in Melbourne because the clients I was seeing day after day had pain management programs that weren't helping them at all. They would do the program and then come out at the end no better off. I also saw doctors and physios who had no idea of how to treat pain once it had become chronic.

The worst case I saw was a receptionist called Amanda who suffered from lower back pain. She was in her mid-thirties and had undergone surgery to fix the problem. The surgery hadn't worked, and by the time I saw her, she was worse off than she had been before the operation. Amanda's doctor had just certified her unfit for work because of her pain. Being stuck at home had made her depressed and in desperation, she had completed a pain program that hadn't helped at all. Before all this, Amanda had been really active and had loved life. I met Amanda at her workplace so that I could get a sense of the physical surroundings with the hope that we could get her back to work. I could see the hope in Amanda's eyes when we spoke. She was desperate to get some normality back.

When Amanda described her pain program to me, I could see that it lacked all of the fundamental elements that we used in the UK to make these programs successful. Worst of all, the insurance company had paid thousands of dollars for the program. I talked to Amanda and gave her some suggestions that would help. She and I then talked to her doctor so that we were all on the same page. We set out a return-to-work plan and before long, she was back at work doing light duties. Best of all was the sense of accomplishment that I could see in her when I visited her at work. She embraced my strategies and they had changed her life.

Working back in Melbourne was an eye-opener. When I was in London, some of the cutting-edge research in pain theory was being done at the very hospital I worked at. There was a greater understanding of what chronic pain was and how it should be treated. Melbourne was still in the very early stages of this understanding. Every day, I saw people in need, and I saw cases like Amanda's where people were being let down and suffering because they couldn't find the right solution.

The difference between the old me and the new me was that now I knew how these people felt. I had been where they were not that long ago. I also knew how vital it was for them to get appropriate advice for a long-term solution. I thought about setting up my own pain physiotherapy service.

While it was good to dream about my pain clinic nirvana, the reality was that I needed to get some capital behind me. I had depleted my savings buying a second-hand car and paying for the insurance and registration. I also needed to continue my own healing journey and pace myself with realistic time-frames for my dreams.

In the meantime, I used every opportunity to get the lay of the land in terms of the treatment of chronic pain. I also had to develop a method that used all the best practices from the pain clinic in London, but add my own experiences into the mix, and then combine the whole lot into a program that people could take away with them.

In London, patients were expected to attend the clinic every day but I knew that this wasn't necessary for everyone. I envisaged an after-hours clinic so that I could continue my day job. An evening clinic would not only allow me to offer a physiotherapy service to pain patients, but encourage their family and carers to participate as well. The support that I had received from friends and family in the aftermath of the attack had been vital to my recovery. I wanted to encourage similar support networks with my patients.

Through my job helping people return to work, I noticed patterns in the treatment of chronic pain around Victoria.

The most striking thing was that most of the sufferers I met had no understanding of managing pain once it moved from the acute stage (within the first three months) into the chronic stage (longer than three months).

A typical example of this was a guy I met called Stefan. He was a house painter in his mid-forties who had hurt his back on the job. By the time the insurance company brought me in on the case – nine months after the initial injury – Stefan was still having physio three times a week but there had been no improvement in his pain levels. I met Stefan and his supervisor at a house they were painting. The first thing I noticed about him was that his pain was obvious. As we spoke, he seemed uncomfortable and he regularly put his hands on his hips and massaged his lower back – the universal action of back pain suffers. He walked with the shuffle of a much older man. The most obvious thing about Stefan was his frustration. He was on light duties, and he kept talking about how nothing was working.

'The pain's still there,' he said over and over. 'There must be something else wrong.'

I had seen copies of Stefan's X-rays and MRI results and nothing else had shown up. Stefan was still seeing his doctor once a fortnight. He described how his physiotherapist used heat packs and massage in the thrice-weekly treatments. Stefan was diligent about completing the regular walks that his physio had prescribed. He had been told to walk until it was too painful and then stop. He also completed some basic daily stretches.

'Has anyone explained to you why you still have the pain?' I asked him.

'No, they just said that there is still something wrong,' Stefan replied.

This is so wrong, I thought. Here was this poor guy who just wanted to get on with his life, and his health care professionals were subjecting him to a treatment that after nine months had shown no sign of working.

I spent time with Stefan and gave him an understanding of why his pain might be persisting. I told him that his solution lay in focusing on improving his physical capacity, rather than merely concentrating on reducing his pain. If he changed the focus, even if the pain levels remained the same, his life would automatically be improved because he was doing more. The flow-on effect from this was that he would then begin to feel the pain less because he was fitter and stronger and busier. His focus would shift from being predominantly on the pain to being predominantly on his life.

'That makes sense,' said Stefan with a hint of hope in his eyes.

'If you alter your perception of your pain and learn to manage it yourself, you can get your life back,' I told him.

Stefan's doctor was like most doctors that I meet; they are always willing to listen to someone who might have a solution to their patient's chronic pain. Meeting Stefan's physiotherapist was a different matter. He was resistant to my suggestion that, because of the lack of progress, he should reduce the hands-on sessions and teach Stefan to self-manage his condition.

A good therapist will assess a patient and have a fairly clear idea of how many treatments will be needed for improvement. Some conditions – like knee reconstructions – will require six to nine months of therapy. These start with treatments up to three times a week in the first month or two, and then gradually reduce to one treatment a week with an exercise regime to promote self-management. Most other conditions or injuries do not require that length or intensity of treatment. Whenever I hear of people like Stefan who have had physio treatments three times a week for nine months, I know that the physiotherapist has little understanding of the treatment of chronic pain. Either that or they are trying to cash in on the insurance company payments. I always try and assume the former and give my colleagues the benefit of the doubt.

One way to tell if health care practitioners are genuinely concerned for their clients is that they embrace my suggestions with relief. Their first and foremost desire is for their clients to improve. Stefan's physiotherapist declared that he knew best because he had been treating Stefan for so long. For me, hitting this brick wall was not uncommon.

The last time I met with Stefan was when he had changed to a more proactive physiotherapist and had returned to work with a much better understanding of his condition. He was standing a bit taller, looked fitter, and most importantly, had a smile on his face. A simple switch in his perception and therapy meant that he had progressed more in the three months that I had been involved in his case, than in the nine months following his initial injury.

The more I moved around Melbourne visiting people like Stefan, the more I wanted to set up my own physiotherapy pain clinic to show people there is another way.

VIN'S MOVE TO MELBOURNE

In May 2007, Vin got the opportunity through her company to transfer to Melbourne and grabbed it with both hands. It was a brave move on her part. She had no friends or family in Melbourne except me. It was the first time she had moved out of home, and as the only daughter, she had been wrapped in cottonwool by her parents. While the move pushed her outside her comfort zone, she was thrilled by the opportunity.

Vin wasn't interested in a share house. As well as working, she was studying for her chartered accountancy program and wanted her own quiet space to study. In her ignorance of Melbourne, she signed up for a small one bedroom apartment in a fancy high-rise on St Kilda Road, right next to the Victoria Police complex. What she (and her protective father who loved the idea of her being next door to hundreds of police officers) didn't realise was that the apartment was also within roaring distance of the Grand Prix race circuit.

And boy, did she get a shock, come March.

The noise from the Formula 1 engines whining like mosquitoes on jet-fuelled steroids pierced her walls, and was then accompanied by revving loud enough to make you feel as if you were track side.

The apartment complex had a fifteen-metre swimming pool, a small gym and sauna, and a tennis court. It was a stone's throw from the city centre and Albert Park Lake, and we both grew to love Port Melbourne beach.

I admired it jealously from my parents' place in Wantirna, and visited as often as I could. I was working in Port Melbourne and she lived about fifteen minutes from my work. After work, I would pop by to keep her company and make sure she was all right. We would have dinner. She would cook the veggies, I would cook the meat. Vin and her whole family were strict vegetarians but Vin bent the rules for me to allow me to cook meat in her apartment.

The subject of me sleeping over was a delicate one, despite the fact that I was thirty years old!

When I was letting my parents know that I wouldn't be home – I had to let them know, otherwise they would wait up – I always rang and quickly alluded to an early meeting in the city so that it made sense for me to stay over.

And then I hung up really quickly.

It was weird having Vin live in Melbourne. For almost a year, she had been a voice on the other end of the phone, and now she was here in person every day. In person, her energy was energising to those around her. While I had kept up some regular fitness like using weights at home and jogging around the block, Vin took it to a whole new level.

We started exercising together, jogging around Albert Park Lake and the track around the tranquil Botanic Gardens known as the Tan. I even used the lap pool and the gym in her apartment complex. It was so much better than pounding the streets of Wantirna.

We did fun-runs together, and I even taught Vin how to ride a bike and swim; this was after she decided to enrol herself in the BRW Triathlon without knowing how to do two of the three activities required. Typical Vin – she would just jump into the deep end without thinking too much.

I sometimes wished I could be that carefree.

But not quite as carefree as the day of the triathlon when one of her teammates dropped out and she signed me up without telling me. Taking a leaf out of her book, I said, 'What the heck!' and jumped right in. I finished, but I certainly didn't break any records and had to have a long lie-down at the end. I had knowingly pushed myself and the chronic pain was knowingly letting me know. The days that followed were unpleasant to say the least, but I wasn't going to let that tarnish the fun we had on the day.

But of course once you start spending time with someone, it's not all rosy. We had more than our fair share of arguments. In fact, the running joke was that if we didn't argue, there was something wrong. Vin was spontaneous, and I liked to plan.

She was the dreamer and I was the realist. She'd leave the dishes on the sink, whereas, I needed to have them washed and dried and put away. It was more hygienic that way. Didn't she *know* that? She wanted to go out for dinner, visit friends and then hit the movies – all within a couple of hours. Didn't she *know* that you can't squash three things into a night and still be on time for the movie? What happened to considering the time it takes getting from A to B?

But despite our arguing, I wanted Vin by my side. She was so precious and there certainly was never a dull moment when she was around. With our growing closeness and my sleepovers, we experienced the kind of subtle undercurrent of pressure from our Sri Lankan and Indian families that only a 30-year-old man and his 28-year-old sweetheart can. Everyone wanted our relationship to go to the next level.

Marriage.

Of course we noticed it. Like you notice a sledge hammer. And soon, Vin was on their bandwagon too. When Vin mentioned the *m*-word, I would kind of brush it off. In my mind, there was no rush.

And I also had something I had to do first.

MEETING UP WITH THE GIRLS AGAIN

It was around December 2007 when Anita emailed me and said she was coming to Melbourne. It's hard to judge the tone of an email, but it seemed a little tentative. She wanted to see me. I was glad she contacted me; we all needed closure.

It had never sat well with me that, in the year since I walked out of our shared house with my farewell confined to the bottle of wine and the card I left behind, we hadn't spoken at all. After going through so much, our friendship had been shattered.

Any anger, at what I saw as them turning on me, had dissipated through my therapy sessions. Although we all went through a traumatic event, I got the support and they were the ones left out on a limb. Time and distance had allowed that understanding to grow.

A part of me wanted them to understand that I hadn't done anything wrong by wanting to come home. Without hesitation, I returned Anita's email and organised to meet her at a pub in St Kilda during her stay in Melbourne the following week.

That gave me a week to ponder our parting.

Even though I understood why the girls reacted the way they did at my decision to leave, it turned out that a small part of me was still a little raw and hurt by their actions – the classic difference between head and heart. Above all else, I was really interested in finding out how Anita had seen things. The fact that she had suggested meeting meant that she probably wanted closure to this as well.

Although Vin was now in Melbourne, I didn't take her with me to the pub. While she knew what had gone on between me and the girls in London, I wanted to test the lay of the land before introducing her to Anita. Just in case.

Anita must have felt the same way because when I arrived, she was waiting for me alone.

When our eyes met, Anita stood up and I could tell by her smile that she was here for the same reasons as me: to get closure, and to see what we could salvage from our once-warm friendship.

I let out a breath of relief. I'm not one for conflict.

After settling at the table with a drink each, we spent the first ten minutes in small talk, and then our conversation eased into something like it used to be – chatting about what we were both up to in our lives. Soon we were laughing and joking like old times, both ignoring the elephant in the room. I knew that as soon as the old warmth returned, it was like the circumstances of our parting no longer mattered. What's done is done. I was just glad to get my friend back.

After an hour, we parted, promising to keep in touch.

Months after Anita's visit, Jill arrived in Melbourne. Like Anita, her first contact had been by email. Jill and I agreed to have dinner. She was holidaying with her parents and a friend from the UK. Not blessed with Anita's diplomacy, Jill was more candid, a say-it-like-it-is kind of person. I wondered what her take on our final weeks would be.

At the dinner table, joined by her family, Jill and I worked in tandem to tell the story of how we had met and our share house experience.

'Oh my God, I totally freaked out on that night!' Jill said as she took a sip of her beer.

'Yeah, it was pretty full-on,' I said laconically.

'I couldn't believe how calm you were,' she said. 'I was having a total panic attack.'

I got a sudden insight of what Friday 23 June 2006 was like from a spectator's point of view. It must have been like a horror movie for them all: seeing me with my skin peeling off, our house on fire and blood everywhere. At least I got to go off to hospital. Jill and Anita and Lauren had stayed on in the burnt house and cleaned up my blood. I saw horror on the faces of Jill's parents and friend as we recounted what happened.

'I just couldn't get it out of my mind,' said Jill quietly. 'If it had happened a couple of minutes earlier, I would have been with you on the couch. It could have been me.'

'Lucky you went into the kitchen to help Anita,' I said. 'Who would have thought that making a salad could have potentially saved your life?'

'You know,' said Jill turning to me, 'you were right to go home when you did.'

'I know,' I said, 'but that didn't stop me from feeling guilty for leaving you guys behind.'

'You *needed* to go home,' she said in a voice that brokered no argument.

And those were the words I needed to hear to bring that chapter to a close. No more words were needed. I was so glad to have both my friends back.

THAT SHOCK, THAT KICK AND THAT RING

By mid-2008, Vin was coming to the end of her Chartered Accountancy program. She had been in Melbourne for almost eighteen months. After everything we had gone through, it really was time for the next stage of our relationship. Also, selfishly, it was a chance to get our parents off our back with all their not-so-subtle hints about marriage, babies and settling down.

It had got to the point where my parents were getting blunter in their approaches,

'Don't you think it's time you settled down?' my mother would say as I wandered into the kitchen to get a glass of water.

'We want to see your children before we die,' my father would say as I sat down on the couch to watch TV with the glass of water in my hand.

Vin's family were more interested in the completion of their cultural parental role: to marry off their daughter. Every time she visited her family home in Sydney, she would be surrounded by relatives warning her not to be too old when she had children, and reminding her that all of her friends were getting married and she should too. There were also inquiries from mothers of unmarried sons her family knew.

'They were asking about you for their son,' Vin's mum would say.

'Mum!' Vin would shriek.

In the end, it wasn't the pressure from both our families, but rather my love for Vin that prompted my decision to propose.

I wanted to surprise Vin. While she excelled in her career, in some ways, she was really gullible. I knew she wouldn't be hard to trick into a proposal situation. First, I bought the ring. Naturally and culturally, I couldn't just go into a jewellery store to get it. I had to hunt down a factory-direct warehouse place that I'd heard about from a mate who'd married a couple of months earlier.

'Go to these guys,' said my mate. 'It's a family business and they will make whatever kind of ring you want.'

My mate failed to mention that the factory in Thomastown was in an industrial estate right next to a sexual merchandise shop. I blushed as I scurried past the big windows through which the passer-by was left in no doubt of the wide range of marital aids in stock. I looked the other way. My mission was to get the most important pre-marital aid – the engagement ring. In the end, I chose a ring with Vin's favourite stone, a blue sapphire, flanked by a diamond on each side.

Then I came up with the perfect idea to surprise Vin.

My friend Chan was visiting from London. He was staying in a hotel in the city and I quickly elicited his help. I was working on the manuscript for this book so I told Vin that I wanted to take some photographs for the book, of me playing the guitar. It would give you, the reader, a visual picture of my rehab. She agreed to come along and help. I said Chan would be there as well to take a few pictures.

Meanwhile, I told Chan to meet us at Federation Square so that we could all walk together to the Botanic Gardens. Once we were there, on cue, Chan would *see something interesting* and wander off to look at it and that would be my moment.

I would propose, and Chan would swing around with camera and capture the moment of surprise on Vin's face forever.

In hindsight, it would mean taking my best mate to my proposal, but I didn't let small details like that interfere with my enthusiasm.

On the morning of 28 June 2008, Vin and I got ourselves organised. I gathered my guitar prop, and made sure I grabbed the all-important camera. We set off on our walk to Federation Square to meet Chan.

It was a sunny but crisp winter's morning – the perfect day for a proposal. I was excited because I knew Vin had no idea of what was about to happen. I was about to pull off the biggest surprise ever and I couldn't wait to see Vin's face.

While we were walking, Vin actually started to say that I had better propose to her soon before her parents dragged her back to Sydney. I knew they were empty threats, because she loved me just as much as I did her, but it meant that she *really* had no idea what I had planned. This was going to be one hell of a day for both of us.

At the time, I thought my proposal plan the most romantic idea. In hindsight, there's a touch of Bollywood about it. Picture me: sitting under a tree in the Botanic Gardens playing my guitar, singing (or trying to) the old Elvis favourite 'Can't help falling in love'.

Vin was looking a little startled.

Chan was over by the Yarra pretending he was greatly interested in the muddy brown waters, clutching my camera and ready to swing around to capture our moment.

I dramatically stopped singing.

Put the guitar down.

Whipped from a sitting to a kneeling position.

And I was ready.

I reached into my pocket for the ring box. I opened the box in front of Vin while Chan stood twenty metres away, clicking the camera with the zoom lens.

'Vin, I love you. Will you marry me?' I asked.

It took a while for Vin to register. I think she was in shock. Then, she kicked me. I think it was an excited kick.

'Um, is that your way of saying yes?' I questioned rubbing the side of my chest where her kick connected.

'Yes!' she said, her eyes alight with excitement.

'Good, because I'm not doing this again,' I said picking up my guitar and brushing the dust from my knees.

It was done.

We were engaged.

For a moment, I had a sudden case of: *Anj what the hell have you got yourself into...* But that was short lived. Almost instantaneously, series of memories flashed before me – from the first day I had spoken with Vin, to the day I saw her at Avalon airport, and right to the moment when she said 'yes'. It was then a case of: *Anj, you've just got engaged to the best thing that has ever happened to you...*

I suddenly had that warm, fuzzy, happy feeling that people talk about.

Relief was the predominant sentiment from both sets of parents. Relief was our predominant sentiment too. No more would we get the sledge-hammer hints about our future and having babies before anyone died.

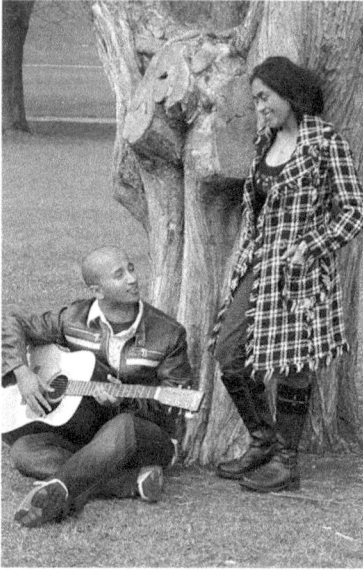

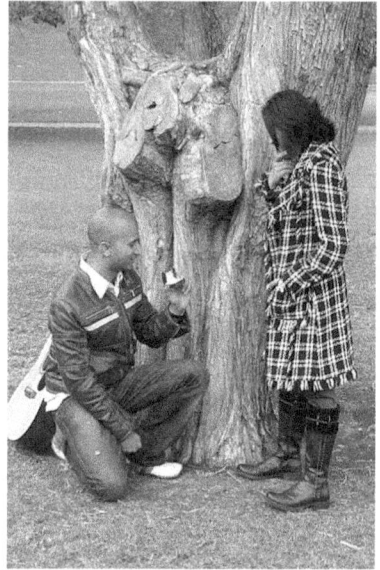

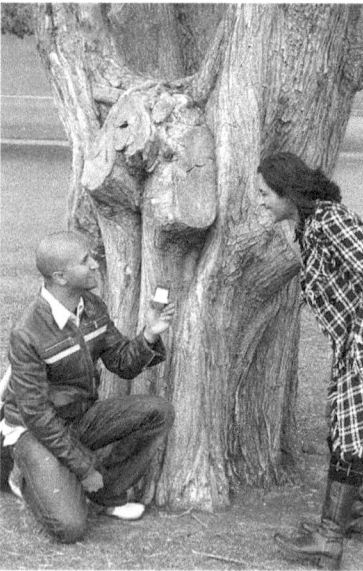

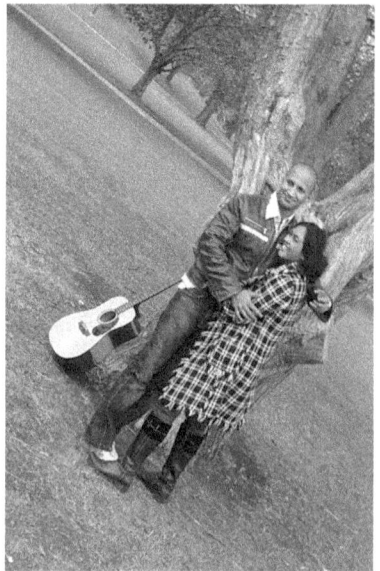

My Proposal

BEYOND PAIN

In August 2008, I was finally in a position to open my pain clinic. It was just months after I had asked Vin to marry me. Vin fully supported my desire to set up a pain management clinic. She knew how important it was for me to help people. Since the petrol bomb attack, I had come to believe that the things I had suffered had been to prepare me for this role. I knew that I was best-placed to help people because I had been on the same pain journey as they. I had pain street-cred.

I wanted to set up my after-hours clinic close to home. I found the perfect location – inside a gym in Ringwood that was willing to rent me some space for my clinic. I loved the idea of setting-up a clinic inside a gym because from the outset, a gym is a place of health and wellbeing which is what I wanted to promote. I could also use the gym's facilities for my clients.

While I ran my clinic two nights a week, I kept my day-job. The beauty of this was that I had a full-time job so I wasn't relying on the clinic for income; instead, I could concentrate on helping others. This meant that I wasn't under any pressure to increase my clinic numbers and I was also able to offer affordable rates to ensure that my services could be accessible to anyone who needed my help.

When the time came to name my clinic, I called it Beyond Pain because I wanted to focus on life beyond the pain.

In my own experience, I knew the importance of looking beyond pain to see what else life had to offer. I didn't advertise widely because I didn't want it to get too big too quickly. Always in the back of my mind, I was conscious of my own pain and limitations. I needed to practice what I preached and pace myself in doing this. As part of my treatment, I ensured that every session had an educational and a practical component.

One of my very first clients was a woman called Lynne who had back and foot problems. She had been referred to me by a physiotherapist who realised that she needed special-ised pain management treatments. Lynne was up-front about her concerns.

'I was told to come and see you,' she said, 'but I don't know what you can do that my other physios haven't done already.' Her scepticism increased when I told her that my program wasn't even hands-on and I would not be doing any manual therapy.

I told Lynne that all she needed was to approach this therapy with an open mind and that I would teach her all the skills she needed to be her own physio. I assured her that this treatment was based on the most current theories in best-practice pain management. She agreed to give it a go.

Lynne was a great client. In just four weeks of following the program set out in Part 3 of this book, she had increased her hours at work, she had tripled the distance she could walk, and reported a significant decrease in her pain levels. She couldn't believe the difference. A practice that I use is to film clients doing physical activities such as walking, standing from sitting and climbing stairs. At the end of the treatment, I film them doing the same activities and then show them the contrasting films for comparison.

It took viewing the films for Lynne to really see just how far she had come. In the early films, she was stiff and slow and struggling to complete the simple tasks. Her confidence mirrored her physical ability. A month later, she did the same tasks with confidence and an ease that she hadn't shown in the first films. While Lynne had noticed an improvement, she couldn't believe the extent until she saw the films together.

After Lynne had completed the program, she left my clinic committed to continue with her strategies and manage her pain on her own. I knew that my program had changed her life. She was a walking example of the reason that I had entered this profession – to help people in need.

Soon, there was a steady stream of people who came to my clinic. The only time I couldn't help someone was when they weren't ready to change. Occasionally, I would get a client who was still too busy looking for a cause to work on a solution, or one who was too focused on their pain that they weren't ready for a solution. Occasionally, I would have people whose pain had become such an integral part of who they were and how they related to those around them, that they were unwilling to believe my program could offer a solution. I always told my clients straight up: 'You don't have to come here if you don't think I can help you.'

The solution always begins and ends in the mind of the client. If they think they can do it, they can. If they think they can't do it, they can't. Luckily for me, most of the people who came to my clinic came because they were genuinely seeking a solution. Those were the people who I could really help.

Helping people is what I wanted to do but I was just one person and I knew my limitations. The idea to put my understandings into a book came from a friend called Nola who developed breast cancer in her mid-forties. Nola had undergone surgery and chemotherapy, but had been left with chronic pain in her chest and arm that had no obvious cause. I spent time with her discussing chronic pain and its causes and treatments. Like so many others, Nola had never heard any of this before and told me that I should write a book about it. I saw the sense in her suggestion and began writing.

Once I started writing, something magical happened. When you start to put your life on paper, it gives you the opportunity to tie up the loose ends, and at the same time reflect, process and digest what has happened. It was both empowering and therapeutic at the same time.

When you have your story on paper, it formalises it. It happened. It was real. It's black and white, which ironically helps you to see the shades of grey in between. I was surprised to see the enormity of the petrol bomb and what it did to me and, by association, the ones I loved. When you experience a trauma, you live from moment to moment initially, then you are so busy taking things one day at a time, that you don't step away to examine the full picture.

When you write it down, things become much clearer. You see yourself.

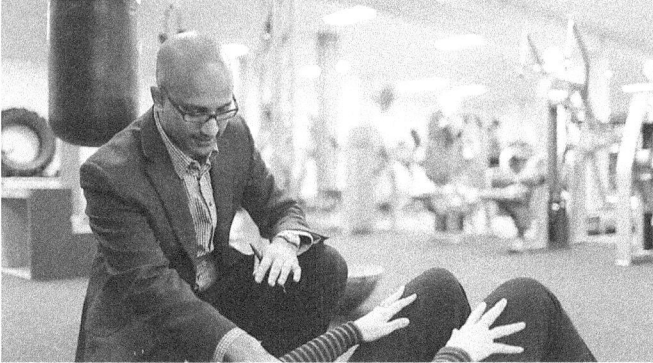

Individualised programs

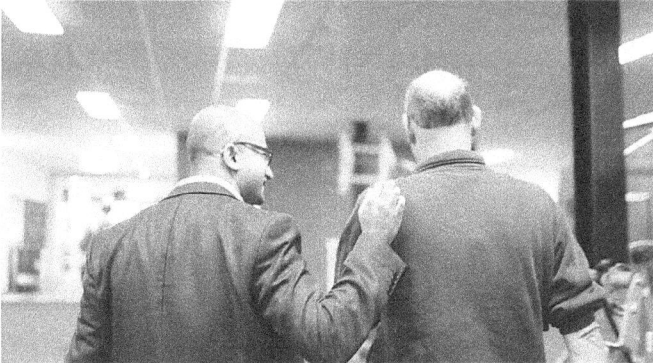

Working together to achieve goals

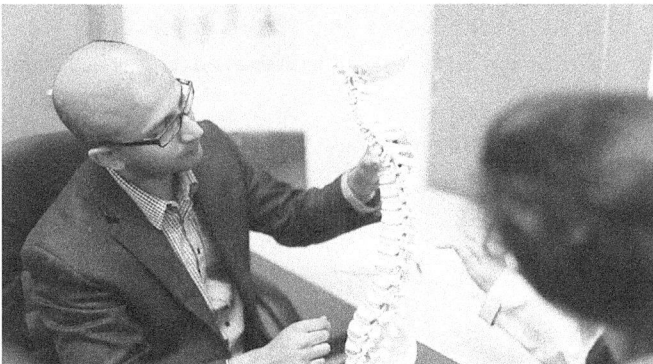

Education is a key component

WEDDINGS AND WHITE HORSES

If I'd ever pictured myself getting married, my vision would have been me in a tuxedo standing in a park with a girl in a white dress saying our vows to a celebrant. We would be surrounded by a hundred family and friends and then have a barbeque afterwards. Beer would be served from bins filled with ice. Salads would be served from bowls on trestle tables, and one of my mates would be working the barbeque filled with sausages and chops. The female Sri Lankan members of the family would fill another trestle table with delicious curries and everyone would have a great time.

Not in a million years would I have ever imagined myself dressed in white coat over a kind of pyjama pants and a maroon-red under-jacket while wearing a white jewelled turban and riding a white horse on the way to my bride. I also never thought my wedding would be a four-day affair with three hundred people and multiple changes of outfits, and that I would do the whole thing wearing satin slippers. I was like a Gujarati Elvis.

Twelve months to the day after my marriage proposal to Vin, I rode on a white horse surrounded by friends and family in traditional Indian and Sri Lankan saris, Punjabi outfits and tuxedos. Vin's family and friends waited at the reception centre while my posse moved slowly up the street towards them. This symbolised the meeting of the two families.

Vin was dressed in a stunning red and white dress trimmed in a sparkling array of jewels. It was the most ornate thing I had ever seen. She looked so beautiful and her usual energetic nature had been replaced by a nervousness that I had never seen before. I quickly made a silly face at her. She laughed and the tension floated away.

After two hours of cultural activities – having our feet painted, walking around a fire, standing on ceremonial pebbles, traditional family wrestling and other things that had to be seen to be believed – Vin and I were finally pronounced husband and wife. It was a wedding of unimaginable proportions, an extravaganza.

After what felt like six thousand photos and a Sri Lankan wedding ceremony so that we were properly married in the eyes of both sets of parents, Vin and I snatched a couple of hours sleep before embarking on our honeymoon the following day – with six friends. Because we had close friends and family come over from the UK for the wedding, we decided to all go to Port Douglas so that we could spend some time together away from the wedding madness. And that was how my cousins Nadie and Sajith, and my best friend Chan came to be on my honeymoon.

It didn't matter that our honeymoon was invaded, because Vin and I had a secret dream of a very different honeymoon. From the moment I left Melbourne all those years ago, I wanted to end my travels in the Himalayas. Vin was keen to help me realise my dream and we made a vow to save up and have our real honeymoon in the foothills of Everest.

For me, it was like coming full circle. I had been through such an incredible journey from leaving home a naïve young man, to coping with a collapsed lung, then the petrol bomb attack, and now the chronic pain with which I was left. Everest base camp stood like a victory beacon, the ultimate goal, the top of the world. For me, it was the epitome of living life beyond my pain.

We just had to save up enough to get there.

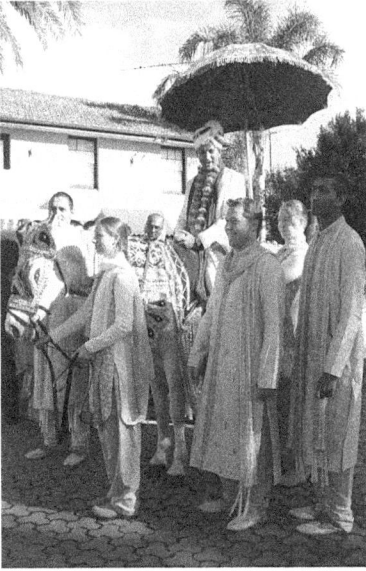

Riding on a horse

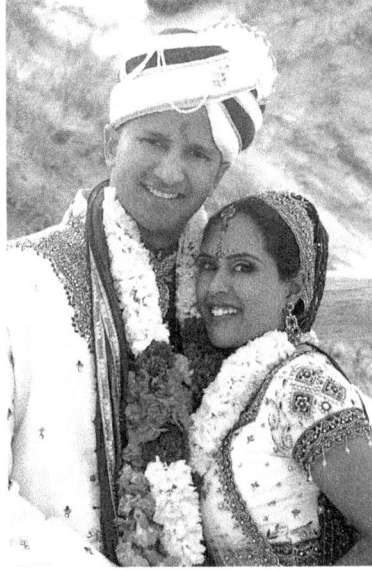

Vin and I at Cronulla Beach

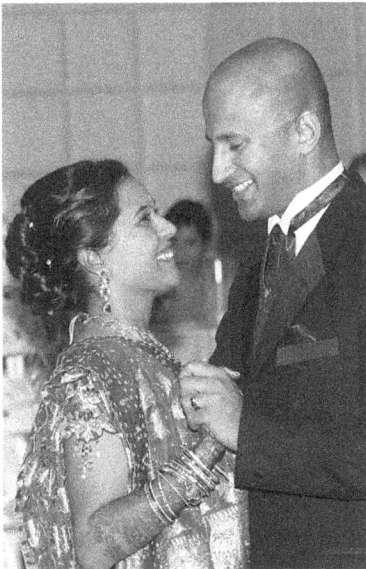

Vin and I at the reception

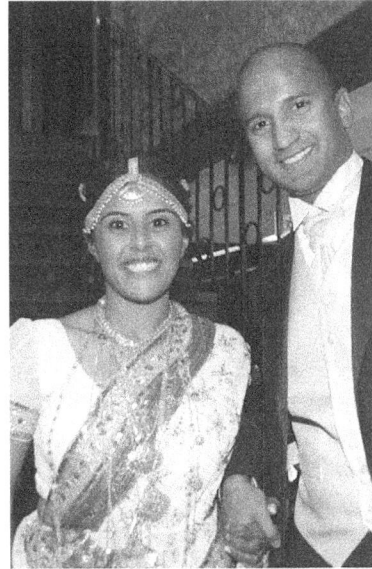

Vin in a traditional Sri Lankan bride's outfit

ON TOP OF THE WORLD

Known as one of the world's most dangerous runways, the landing strip in Lukla is notoriously short, but that's not the problem. The problem is that it ends in a stone wall, which meant that, if the tiny twin engine Otter-type plane doesn't stop in time, it will crash. If that wasn't worrying enough, there were no safety demonstrations on the plane, just a lolly to suck on to make your ears pop and ear plugs of cotton wool so your ears don't get blocked. The day before Vin and I landed, a plane had crumpled its nose against the wall. Thankfully, our forty-minute flight from Kathmandu ended with our plane landing safely.

And that's how our honeymoon in the Himalayas began, just over a year after we got married. At 2860 m above sea level, Lukla marked the beginning of an eight-day hike to the base camp of Mt Everest. Eight days up the incline, four days back downhill. Aside from helicopters, the hike was the only way in and out.

In preparation Vin and I had done some hiking locally back in Melbourne, particularly the 1000 steps at the base of Mt Dandenong. We had also done some running and swimming to make sure our fitness was as good as it could be to complete this trek. But glimpsing the huge mountains rising well above the clouds from the plane, I got a niggling feeling that maybe we should have trained a bit harder.

As we collected our luggage from the plane, it dawned on

me that getting to the Mt Everest base camp was not just a personal pursuit, but now also a professional one. It was a chance to show my clients that with the right attitude and training, you can achieve your goals, no matter how large or small, and no matter what you have gone through.

My message wasn't: *hey, look at what I have achieved, but rather: don't give up, there is a way.*

Most of my clients ended up with chronic pain, not through a random attack like mine, but because they had lifted something at work or strained themselves cleaning the bath at home. They didn't want to climb to the Mt Everest base camp, they just wanted to return to doing day-to-day chores without a constant struggle. I just hoped that my atypical story wouldn't seem too removed from the everyday chronic pain sufferer's story.

Pain is pain, no matter what the source.

It's what you do about it that counts.

Dealing with it is all about setting meaningful goals, great and small, and working through the highs and lows towards achieving them. At first, the journey may feel challenging but, hey, it took me five years to set foot in the Himalayas; and it all started with an exercise bike next to my hospital bed.

Small steps.

'Vin, I can't believe we made it here.' I grabbed Vin's shoulders and shook vigorously with a grin from ear to ear.

'I know. Let the adventure begin,' she replied, enthusiastic as ever.

The great unknown for all who attempt trekking in the Himalayas is the altitude. At 4500 m above sea level, the oxygen levels are about half of what we have in our everyday lives; our destination was 5365 m. Shortness of breath and headaches are common at this altitude. The locals don't suffer from any of the symptoms; their bodies have adapted to their environment. They have more red blood cells, their blood carries more oxygen, and hence works more efficiently.

Even though Mt Everest isn't visible from Lukla, I had to pinch myself; there were times when I doubted whether I would ever make it to this place. Until now, I had been close, but always pulled away at the last minute: the collapsed lung, the petrol-bomb, chronic pain and going home to Australia. But if you want something bad enough, there is a way. If my journey up until this moment had taught me anything, that was it.

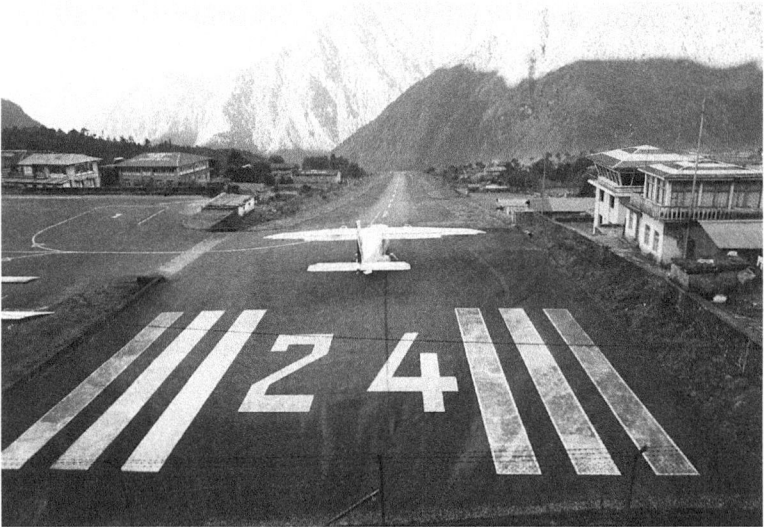

The dangerous runway at Lukla Airport

There is a way.

Vin shared my dream of Mt Everest and was as excited as I was, but there was a difference. For her, it was an exciting adventure, but for me, it was more of a destiny thing. If I could do this, I could prove to myself that anything *is* possible.

Our group of trekkers included some seasoned travellers who had done the Inca trails and Kilimanjaro. In all there were six of us from Australia, two guys from Sweden, an educator from England, a dairy farmer from Canada and a 58-year-old breast cancer survivor from America. We all met up in Kathmandu with our head guide, Ram, and flew in on the tiny twin-engine plane together. At Lukla airport, we met our assistant guides and our porters. For the next two weeks, we would be spending every waking moment together. I got a really good vibe from the group and so did Vin.

While Kathmandu was busy and dusty, Lukla was crisp and fresh. The sky was cornflower blue with white cotton-candy clouds. In the distance, a shark-fin shaped mountain of grey rock, Kongde Ri, towering some 6187 m, stood out among all the others. Ram told us that it was regarded as a holy mountain by the locals and that it was one of the most difficult to climb. Seeing the Holy Mountain made me excited for the mountains to come.

The trek began straight after breakfast at a local Lukla guesthouse. Vin and I donned our small backpacks and handed our larger backpacks to the porters. I had never seen anything like it. The porters loaded up with bags and each porter carried two big backpacks, which probably weighed around fifteen kilos each. And off they went. Even at this lower altitude, the air was noticeably thinner, but the porters didn't seem to notice. We, carrying our five kilogram packs, struggled more than they did. They quickly disappeared with our luggage, off to the lodge where we would stay that night.

The local houses in Lukla were mud and brick and the one thoroughfare was dirt. Locals had set up stalls to line the tourist route catering both to those wanting local trinkets and those ill-prepared for the cold. Knitted beanies, puffy jackets and sleeping bags were snapped up by tourists just in case. It was October, which is technically autumn in the Himalayas. The region doesn't really have a summer; the seasons go from winter to the monsoon to autumn and back to winter.

Children played happily in the front yards and steered clear of tourists; most vanished when cameras were pointed at them. An occasional cheeky exception stuck out a little hand and asked for chocolate. Vin and I handed out some of the little koala key rings that we had brought especially for such occasions. The kids were delighted but puzzled. Through Ram's translations, they soon understood that the animal on the key ring was from Australia.

A journey of a thousand miles begins with a single step. Our journey wasn't quite that long, but our first steps through Lukla marked the beginning. Surrounded by locals selling food and wares, our guide, Ram, his assistants and our fellow trekkers, we made our way through the little village and into the national park that provided a gateway to the Himalayas in the form of a white concrete arch with a message telling us to have a nice trek.

The first leg of the journey was a slight decline. It would be the only respite our calves would have. That night, my back and my arms also gave me grief. I felt sharp little electric shocks running down my arms. It was like ants with tiny sharp claws were marching up and down my arms. I had first felt these shocks when I was doing rehab, a couple of weeks after the petrol bomb attack. The feelings would come and go, and I had learnt to adapt to them. This buzzing throb in my arms would get much worse if I was stressed, and it could be exacerbated by strenuous exercise. Over time, I had learnt to read this feeling. If I felt that it was stress that was causing it, I used relaxation and deep-breathing techniques. If it was caused by physical exertion, I used stretching and rubbed the affected areas with a soothing cream.

To add to the pain I was experiencing, the surgical scar from my collapsed lung joined in on the action. It felt like there was broken glass rubbing against my skin. I got Vin to use the butt of one of the walking sticks and poke the sore spot in my back.

'Aaahhh, that feels good,' I whispered as I rocked my head back and closed my eyes with relief.

I had always known that this wouldn't be easy. I guess at this point, I had two choices: keep going or give up. And, there was no way I would even think of giving up. No way! Besides, I was confident that my body would hit a stride and adapt to what I was asking of it.

By the second day, it was all uphill. Vin and I woke up in our humble room, thankful that we had brought good-quality sleeping bags. The walls of the lodge were thin and insulation unheard of. There was no sound-proofing and by the next morning, we all knew the snorers.

I was pleased with the way I had handled the initial hike, even though it was downhill. In the thin mountain air, I hadn't struggled much. Vin and I kept up a good walking pace, and I hadn't noticed any worsening of the chronic pain in my back – there was too much else to look at and too much to take in. Distraction is a good tool in the treatment of chronic pain, and I had the most amazing distractions around me.

As we began our second day, the sun was out and it soon took away the chill of the morning. Clouds drifted across the sky, but when they cleared, the mountains they'd been hiding took our breath away. Occasionally, Ram told us about mountains we passed or pointed things out, but the rule of thumb seemed to be 'less talking, more walking'. In this thinner air, we needed all the oxygen we could process

172   BEYOND PAIN

just to keep moving.

I had a stopwatch function on my watch and made sure that Vin and I stopped at least every twenty minutes for a minute or two to catch our breath and drink some water. Pacing was really important, especially for me. The recommended water intake on the trek was four litres a day each. This amount helped prevent the common altitude headaches most people suffered at these heights. It also helped prevent dehydration. We were rugged up, but sweating with the exertion. There would be no showers for the whole trip. Apparently, having a hot shower in such cold weather wasn't good for your system. I imagined that we would all smell like yaks by the end of the trek. Yaks are native to this part of the world. They look like big hairy buffalo, and are used for carrying cargo. Due to their hairiness and their thick skin, they only live at high altitudes in relatively cold climates. In the Himalayas, they are everywhere.

Sometimes the position of our track let us see up ahead, and the journey or the incline was scary. Pine trees lined the trail of green and spread out for kilometres. The upward sloping landscape was dotted with lodges and small farms. The pristine environment was untainted by smog or pollution; air had never smelt so good.

In what must be the greatest linguistic irony, the locals refer to these mountainous treks as 'the Nepalese flats'. It could be irony, or it could be a form of Nepalese tourist propaganda: 'It's a little bit steep; but then a gentle flat,' was Ram's favourite and oft-repeated mantra. Of course, there was no *flat*, and rarely was it gentle.

Every couple of hours, we stopped at a village that consisted of livestock – cows, goats and chickens – and maybe a hundred locals manning stalls selling water, food and trinkets. We were told to eat vegetarian on the trip because the meat came from Lukla and was carried up the mountains by porters or on the back of cows or yaks. That meant that it spent a lot of time not refrigerated. Salads were off the menu too. Vegetables, fried rice, noodles and soup were the main fare, anything that cooked away any harmful bacteria. Vin and I had taken chocolate bars to snack on at night to replenish the energy that was sapped by the high altitudes. It was pretty cool *having* to eat chocolate for your health.

Everywhere we hiked, there were colourful prayer flags tied overhead from tree to tree. I hadn't seen them before, but Ram told us that the writing on them was traditional Buddhist prayers. Locals had been stringing them up like this for a thousand years. They brought good luck and protected the people. Vin and I bought a couple and planned to string them up when we reached the Mt Everest base camp.

Suspension metal-meshed walking bridges carried us over the rushing Dudh Kosi River as we made our way up the emerald-green terrain. The bridges were usually about half a kilometre long and stretched high above the valleys below. They went down in a gentle arc, making the first part of the crossing downhill, then swept upwards so that you noticed the second half by the tension in your calf muscles.

The journey was so winding that we crossed the Dudh Kosi River five times in one day. The roaring of the white waters crashing over rocks could be heard from miles away. We shared the suspension bridges with oncoming yaks – five yaks to one farmer. There were two choices when confronted by a yak pack coming towards you. If you weren't too far across the suspension bridge, it was easier to retreat. If you were halfway across the bridge, even if you wanted to retreat, you couldn't outrun the yaks in the thin air and they would catch up with you. The only option was to cling on to the cyclone-wire side and pray while the yaks went past almost crushing you. You also had to try and keep your backpack away from the big yak horns just in case the horn caught on your strap and you ended up being part of the yak caravan going the other way.

We used porters rather than yaks because the porters earned a living from carrying tourists' luggage. If we had used a small herd of yaks, then the money would all go to the one family that owned the herd and not be spread around. Ram explained that to us. Ram was around 50 years old and I guessed that he would have to be really fit since he told us that he had been leading this trek for fifteen years. *Slowly, slowly catch a monkey* – that was his other favourite saying. Speed was not the key to trekking, not in this altitude. I heard him say it often enough to consider repeating it to my clients back at the pain clinic. We only walked around seven kilometres each day, but at this altitude, it took us about seven hours. It's hard to imagine one kilometre taking one hour. Back home, hiking in the Dandenong Ranges, we can do three or four kilometres in an hour. Here, if you tried to go any faster, you would get an instant altitude headache.

Ram had prepared us for the fact that this beautiful terrain wouldn't last. As the oxygen dwindled and the temperatures dropped, the conditions became too harsh for most forms of vegetation.

Even in the most remote parts of our climb on the second day, we saw concrete stupas – Buddhist structures, sometimes containing a relic or a statue of Buddha inside them. These and the omnipresent prayer flags were a reminder that this region was filled with devotees of the same faith as me. It was nice to see these symbols as part of the land. I have never considered Buddhism as a religion, but rather a way of life. These prayer flags and stupas were a way of life for the people around me, not showy, but part of the landscape.

The people we met were gentle and kind, always smiling. Most homes were stone or wooden huts with no electricity and no motorised transport. It was like stepping back in time to pioneer days for us, but the locals were living contented lives in this harsh beauty. It really made us think about our reliance back home on electricity and TV. Here, life was simple. At night, we trekkers played cards at the lodges until the generators were turned off at 9 pm. Bedtime came straight after that. Exhaustion after walking all day was felt by all of us. It was a simple life of activity and rest.

The river that raged and crashed on the second day, provided the most amazing waterfalls by the fourth day. Sometimes they were so huge that you couldn't see the top or the bottom. The amount of water was a testament to how much snow must be melting thousands of metres above us. Sometimes the terrain was an upward-sloping path, and other times, the path turned into rocky steps that needed to be carefully negotiated. We would climb for about twenty metres, and then need a break.

It was good to have my wife as a companion – we spurred each other on. Sometimes I wanted to collapse with exhaustion and sometimes she did. 'Let's just get to that big rock over there,' I would say. 'Now we can just get to that next big rock...' That's how it went. The notion of one step at a time became very real for us. One foot in front of the other.

An incredible phenomenon that we saw were thousands of prayers scratched neatly into rock faces in the middle of nowhere along our walking path. They were etched in neat rows four times my height. How people got up this high to create them beggared belief. But then again, we regularly saw porters carrying hundred-kilo loads stride past us not even out of breath while we puffed and panted carrying our few kilo day packs. These mountains were a place that defied physical laws.

We learnt a lot about patience from Ram. And politeness. He was a humble guide and taught us much about the local customs. He also had a sense of fun and would sometimes challenge some of the other trekkers to a race. One thing that he did amazed me. A trekker in our group got sick while we were trekking. He couldn't catch his breath and had to stop. Ram ran about a kilometre ahead to catch the lead porter to retrieve the man's backpack, then ran back again without even puffing. We could walk fifteen metres and be short of breath in this altitude and here was Ram running a kilometre uphill and looking like he was out for a short stroll. It certainly made us think about what these mountain people were made of and how different their adaptations must be. Ram and the other guides were so polite that they never made us feel bad about our physical shortcomings.

Our trek was full of surprises. In the middle of nowhere, we would come across quite large towns. It was incredible that the residents of these remote places could only come in and out of town by walking or by helicopter. Most of them couldn't afford a helicopter ride, so walking was a way of life. We were told that for these locals to get to Kathmandu, it was around a fourteen-day walk. Merchants, farmers and porters would make the journey regularly. Very little of the staples were locally produced and there was only one way in – the rocky path that we had just climbed.

From above, the patchwork of coloured roofs of the town's lodges dotted the green of the mountain side while low hanging clouds made the sky disappear. By now, we were so high up that we were in the clouds and sometimes, mist blocked out the landscape completely. As Ram had promised, the trees became sparse shrubs. The occasional yellow or red flower would break the olive-green carpet.

Little white stone cottages of the local Sherpa people, dotted the landscape as the terrain thinned. They looked like the pictures little kids draw of cottages with a door in the centre and two higher windows, sitting like eyes. The obligatory chimney stuck out of the roof.

By the fifth day, there were no trees at all. The landscape was a carpet of grasses, shrubs, flowers and coloured leaves. I, Vin and the woman from America had taken our place at the back of the group each day. One of the assistant guides, Ram's right-hand man Tashi, hummed Nepalese songs to help keep us going. Breaking the trek into eight days meant smaller, more achievable goals. One foot in front of the other. I was okay; my breathing was fine and my back felt fine. My feet were sore at the end of each day and so were my shoulders, but then again, so were everybody else's. I had decided before the trip that any symptoms that I felt, I would just deal with them. I knew that if I paced myself, rested regularly, and did things sensibly, I would make it.

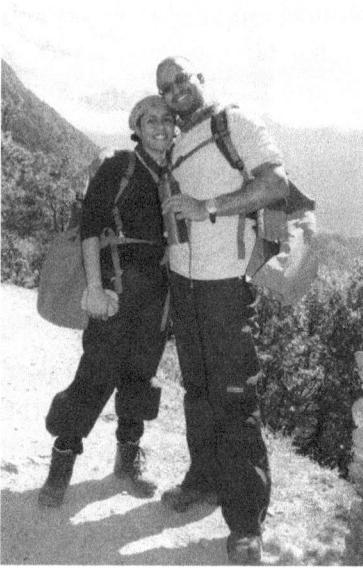

Trekking on day 1

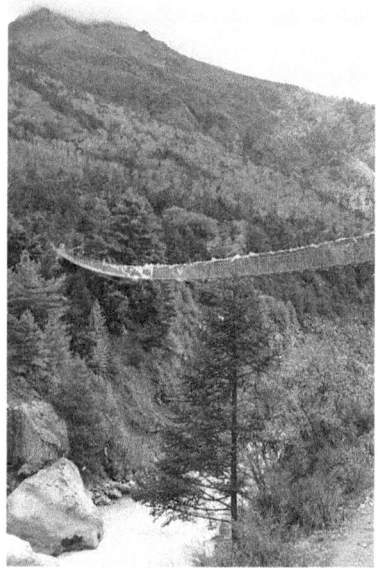

One of many suspension bridges

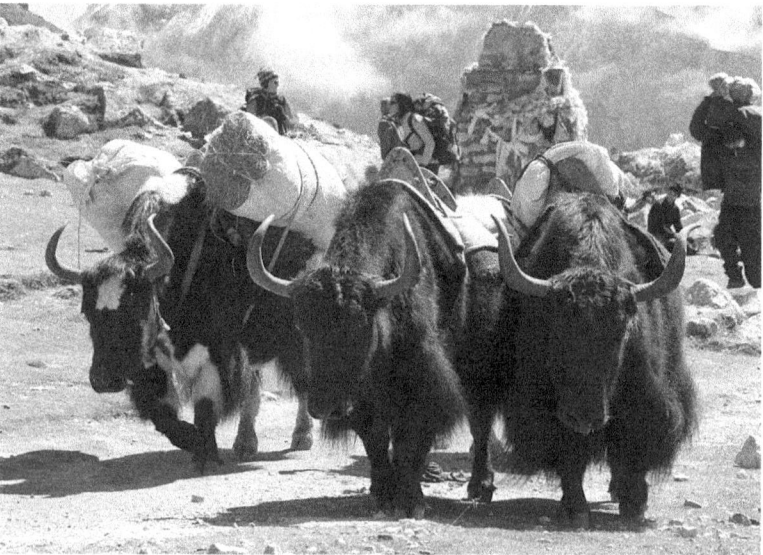

Fully laden yaks on the trail to the base camp

I was methodical in my quest. I kept using the timer to make sure I had regular breaks every twenty minutes. Vin and I each took two one-litre bottles of water each morning, drank them by lunch, then replaced them for the afternoon journey. I made sure that I stretched each morning and night, and I tried to get a decent night's sleep.

At every town we hiked through, there were signs telling us how high we were above sea level. Ram had warned us that from 4000 m upwards, the air would get significantly thinner. The guides carried bottles of oxygen in case anyone got really sick. We all heard stories of people getting altitude sickness so badly that they had to turn around and go home. We'd even seen one of our group have to do the same thing. I was potentially more susceptible to it because I had suffered a collapsed lung in the past, but I pushed any thoughts of this out of my mind. I didn't want to think that I couldn't make it.

Turning back was not an option.

On the seventh day, while travelling from Dimboche to Lobuche, we hiked up a steep rocky pass known as Thukla Pass. There we came upon carefully piled stones draped with prayer flags and ornaments. Ram told us that they were memorials built by locals to commemorate family and friends who had died while on expeditions to the summit of Mt Everest. While tourists who died on Mt Everest always made the news, these mounds of stones reminded us that the locals were equally at risk. Ram told us the story of a Sherpa called Babu Chiri, who had summited Mt Everest eleven times. On his final fatal trip, he had been filming the climbing party when he slipped down a crevice and was killed.

These square stone piles, set in a rocky outcrop like a line of gate keepers, were strangely inspiring. The people they commemorated had made the climb that we were taking many times, and not with the luxury of just carrying the small daypacks that we carried. The memorials were also a stark reminder of the dangers of this landscape, even for people who knew it like the back of their calloused hands.

That morning, I had begun to doubt that I would be able to make it. My back was really sore and my neck was really tight. I even felt a nagging ache in the back of my left calf muscle. It felt like it was deep inside, and as I put my hand on my calf to give it a rub, I noticed an unusual tough lump. It was the size of a golf ball, tough but not painful. I put it down to another tight muscle and tried to just massage it out. I was even struggling for breath while I was resting. I had no appetite. Altitude sickness was combining with my chronic pain issues. Vin and I had talked at our lodge before we set off.

'I don't feel a hundred per cent,' I told her. 'I don't know if I can make it today. I can't believe that we've got this far and things are playing up now. If I can't do this, you should still go on.'

'Don't be stupid! I'm not doing this without you.' Vin used her don't-argue tone.

'But we're only a day away. It doesn't make sense for you not to finish it when we're so close. Even if I can't.'

'Don't worry, Anj,' she said, soothingly 'we'll just go slow.'

I searched her face for any shred of doubt. There was none. Her confidence in me was infectious and her moral support was vital. I checked my pulse which was fine and that meant my lungs were fine. If I forced some food down, paced the walk properly and drank plenty of water, I should be fine.

'Okay, let's do it,' I said, grinning. It made me think about what I always tell my clients back at the pain clinic. Challenge your unhelpful thoughts. Pace yourself. Relax with a deep-breathing technique. I did all of those things.

An hour into the walk, the lump in my calf was still there, but my breathing had improved and I felt much better. It was like I had got a second wind. A second chance. Moral support, positive mindset and chocolate had done the trick. My spirits soared along with my sugar levels.

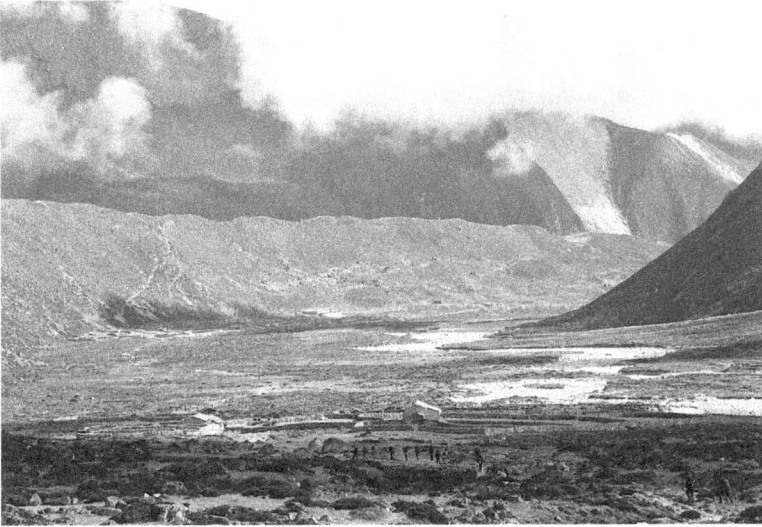
One of many vast desolate valleys

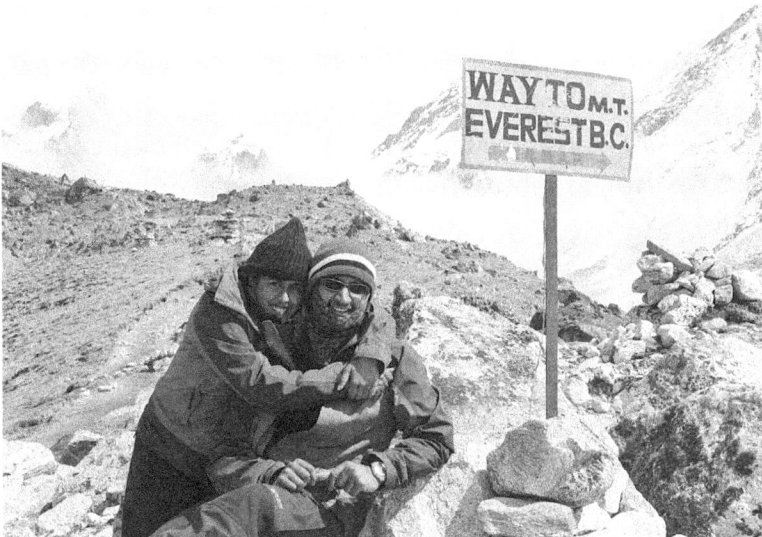
Not far from Base Camp

The higher we got, the more the landscape changed. The carpet of shrubs and grasses gradually vanished and were replaced by rock. The landscape turned from green to grey.

On the morning of the eighth day, we caught our first glimpse of Mt Everest.

We could have seen it earlier from a different vantage point, but the weather had closed in and obscured the view. To look upon the great mountain, albeit a tiny snippet of its peak, was an overwhelming feeling of achievement. I was so close. Base camp was about six hours away.

Looking at the landscape, we might as well have been on the moon. The bleak desolate surroundings were beautiful with their backdrop of the snow-covered Himalayas. All of us felt the humbling effect of smallness in the face of giants. The vastness of the mountains made ants out of us mere mortals. The approach carried its own dangers. Narrow paths with sheer cliff faces on either side meant the possibility of landslides. Ram told us to hurry through. Instead of his normal position at the back of the group, he hurried ahead. 'I'll see you there,' he said, over his shoulder.

'Our guide's just gone off on us,' I said to Vin. 'This can't be good.'

Vin's eyes widened as she took in the sound of small rocks tumbling down the cliffs, and Ram's diminishing back disappearing down the track ahead. She said a rude word or two, grabbed my hand and hurried on in the thin freezing air.

We walked the narrow winding track between the crumbling mountains for about two hours. We all breathed a sigh of relief when we reached the other side.

On the barren plain of the home-stretch to base camp, the cornflower-blue sky was suddenly overtaken by a cloud mass that rolled in through the valley towards us like a tidal wave gathering momentum. It rose kilometres and blotted out the sun and blue sky backdrop with freezing white. Bringing with it, snow and sleet and freezing temperatures, the cloud moved past like a slow-moving spaceship. It was cold enough to freeze camera batteries so that it couldn't be recorded. I had never felt cold like it. It was extraordinary how quickly conditions could change. Sunny to freezing. Clear to dangerous.

In the middle of an unseasonal snow storm, we finally reached our destination.

Mt Everest base camp. We made it!

Being on the rooftop of the world almost brought tears to my eyes, and I wasn't the only one. Plenty of my fellow trekkers clearly felt the same, looking around, blinking away tears as they gazed out onto majestic snow-covered mountains from the desolate base camp. I had come so far. I had finally made it, beaten the odds. Vin was by my side. We had done it together. She knew how much this meant to me, but at the same time, she was happy that she had climbed to the base camp of Mt Everest for herself. That's what the mountain does to you.

There was a huge boulder adorned with prayer flags and graffiti telling us that we were 5364 m above sea level, and that before us, it had been visited by Mizza, Roshan, Lisa and Morgan, among others. From the remoteness of our journey, the base camp was crowded with people; about fifty milled around in the freezing cold marvelling at the conclusion of their own journeys.

We couldn't see Mt Everest's summit from the base camp. It was another 3500 m above where we were, and to get there was an impossible journey for most people. Even though it seemed close, the journey is dangerous because above 6000 m, the oxygen becomes so thin that you need oxygen tanks. Added to this, the temperature drops dramatically and the weather conditions are changeable and perilous. We had glimpsed how quickly things could change with the rolling cloud of sleet and snow. Up higher, things were worse.

For us mere mortals who didn't want to risk our lives or spend exorbitant amounts of money – sometimes hundreds of thousands of dollars – we were satisfied to bask in Mt Everest's foothills.

The time for reflection and photographs was cut short because of the extreme cold. I had one thing to do before we left this place. One of the other guys in the group and I began piling some big stones, one on top of the other, to make an amateur version of the monuments we had seen along the way. When one pile was finished, we made a second pile about a metre away. Between the two piles, we strung a single strand of coloured prayer flags.

As we all took a moment to look down at this symbol of our journey, the flags flapped in the bitter cold wind. Our simple mounds stood among others of a similar nature. The little shrine symbolised the respect we felt for the land and the people. I secretly hoped that it would act as a prayer for our safe return from this desolate yet beautiful place.

HAPPILY EVER AFTER

For me, climbing to the Mt Everest base camp was the beginning. Since then, Vin and I have trekked the Inca Trail and explored Machu Picchu. If I had thought that Mt Everest was the pinnacle back in 2010, my life would have been poorer for it.

Life is about always looking for the next challenge, the next way to find out more about what you're made of. To test your mettle.

We got back from South America at the end of May, and to our surprise, Vin found out she was pregnant mid-June.

Around the twenty-week mark in the pregnancy, Vin wasn't the only one getting ultrasounds. The lump in my left calf that I'd first felt while trekking the Himalayas hadn't gone away. It hadn't bothered me, so I had done nothing about it, but Vin was worried and she made me see a doctor. Before I knew it, I was getting ultrasounds too. Vin's were exciting. Mine were worrying. I played down my concerns, particularly when I spoke to Vin. The last thing I wanted was for her to be stressed.

The doctor suspected a tumour and sent me to one of the best surgeons in Melbourne who confirmed it.

'It looks like a benign tumour,' he told me, analysing at the scans. 'We see them all the time. It will continue to grow slowly. If you want, you can come back in six months when it's uncomfortable and we can remove it. Or I am happy to book you in for surgery now.'

'I don't want a tumour growing inside me,' I said, shuddering at the thought. 'Better out than in.'

My long-suffering father came with me for the procedure a few days later. I didn't want Vin coming with me considering she was in the third trimester of her pregnancy. And because hospitals are magnets for sick people, I also didn't want her catching any hospital bugs. My instinct told me that my decision to have the tumour removed was the right one.

Dad kept a brave face, either that or he wasn't worried at all. I guess after all the procedures he'd accompanied me to in the past, me getting a lump removed from my leg was like a walk in the park.

I got the lump taken out on the Thursday, went home that night, went back to work the next day and didn't give it much more thought. I had a full work schedule and a pregnant wife to take care of.

A week later, the surgeon rang. 'Anjelo,' he said, 'I've got some bad news.'

'What do you mean?' I asked, confused. I hadn't even expected to hear from the doctor again.

'The tumour isn't benign,' he said. 'I didn't believe the pathology results so I got the tests repeated three times in the lab.'

Feeling floored, I stammered a question about what kind of cancer it was.

'It's a rare cancer called a Leiomyosarcoma. Less than one per cent of population have it. I need you to have a CT scan done immediately to see if it has spread. I'll book you in for tomorrow.'

Vin.

The baby.

Cancer.

'Let me know what time you want me,' I told the doctor. I felt numb. *Why couldn't life just let me be?*

I decided to tell my parents first because they lived just down the road. Vin was at work, and I wanted to tell her in person. This was not something that you can say over the phone.

Maybe my parents were a little more used to my medical emergencies by now, and were both surprisingly calm at my announcement. I was proud of them. And in a way, their calm calmed me.

This was another thing to deal with, one step at a time.

Vin cried when I told her. Then, she googled. Within half an hour, she knew more about it than most.

The next morning it was my turn to cry. I couldn't help it, but I knew that I needed to let it out. It began in a primal way; how could I continue to have weird stuff happen to me. But then it became a sob of acceptance, and after a few minutes, my practical side took over. I wiped the tears and it was back to being focused on what to do next.

What could I do that was helpful?

I decided to wait for the CT scan. No sense getting carried away before we knew something for sure. Also, the prospect of what the scans might find was too scary to think about.

Fortunately, the scans were clear and the cancer hadn't spread to other parts of my body.

I was referred to a cancer specialist and it took about five weeks before I was under the knife again to remove the rest of the cancer. In a way, the wait was almost worse than the diagnosis itself; the worry, the uncertainty, and the different scenarios you end up playing out over and over in your head. Of course, you try and stay focused, but when you get diagnosed with The Big C, sometimes it's not that easy. Then you try a bit of humour, joke about how you're just trying to get some attention because you've missed being in the health limelight, and try and take it as it comes. For me, this worked.

Analysis of the tumour showed that it was so rare that doctors weren't even sure if chemo or radiation therapy would help. *Trust me to be in that less than one per cent category.* Luckily, further biopsies showed no sign of the cancer, but I was told that I would need six-monthly checks just in case.

There are always new things to learn about ourselves, and most learning occurs when we are put to the test. With this new test, I tried to use what I knew worked: maintain my sense of humour and take it all in my stride... or limp as the case may be.

Helping to take my mind off myself was also my heavily pregnant wife and the impending birth of our child. Also taking my mind off myself was the fact that our baby was due on 28 February in a leap year. One day late, and the kid would be doomed to only having a real birthday every four years.

Luckily for Layla, and her future annual birthday parties, she came on her due date. In the blink of an eye (but longer for Vin) I was holding my precious new princess in my arms. It's a feeling that no father can possibly put into words.

Life can be full of miracles.

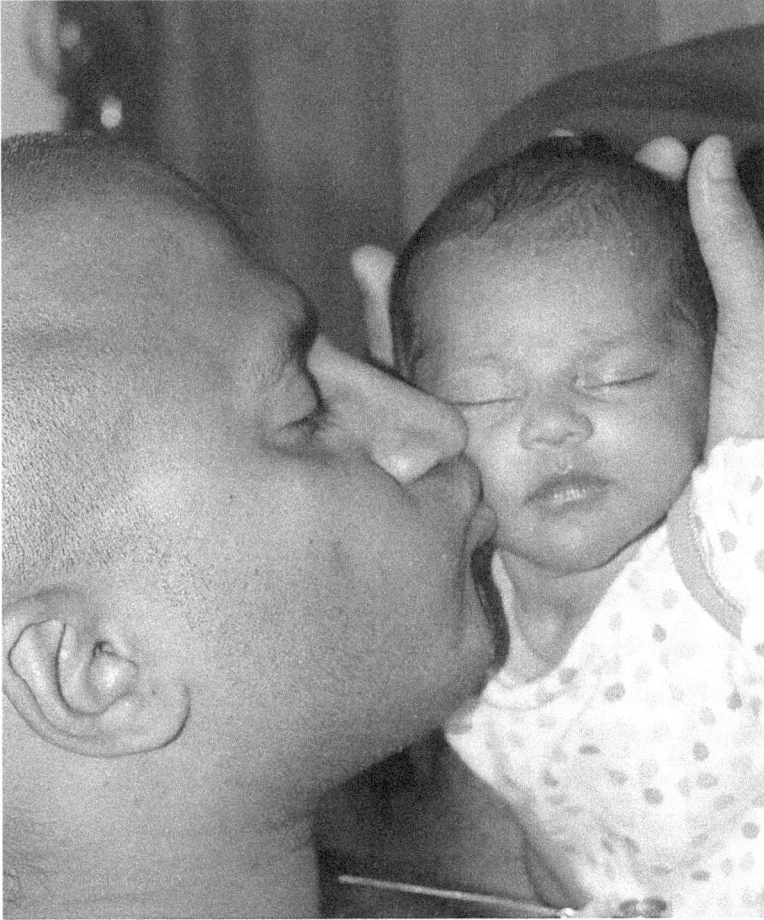

A small miracle

ANYTHING'S POSSIBLE

Aside from completing a personal journey, my hope is that the trek to base camp of Mt Everest can give you hope that anything is possible. It begins with a dream, a purpose, and then the steps to make that dream come true.

Sure there were times when I thought I would never get to the Himalayas: lying in the hospital bed with a collapsed lung; lying in a hospital bed with the skin burnt off my arms and face; and retreating back to Australia. Yes, at those moments, anyone could be forgiven for thinking *that guy won't make it*. But ultimately, it doesn't matter what anyone else thinks. It's what *you* think that matters.

Two thousand years ago, the Greek philosopher Epictetus said, 'It's not what happens to you, but how you react to it that matters.' I love this quote because it is about moving forward. All pain sufferers endure tough times and live through difficulties. That is our baseline. But from there, it is our attitude and our choices that make all the difference. We can choose to let it control us and suffer, or we can choose to take steps to improve our lives.

When you think about it, it's not just about pain, it's about life choices. Do you want to make the most of what you have and enjoy life to the fullest? Do you want to grab life by the horns, or let it slip away, filled with pain and suffering? Do you want to achieve your dreams and maybe show someone else that they too can achieve theirs?

A T-shirt popular in the 1980s carried the simple motto: Choose Life. That is what my story is all about, choosing life, and choosing to live a purposeful life.

Thinking back to those minutes sitting in the upstairs bathtub after the petrol bomb had set me on fire, believing the house to be on fire and believing my death to be imminent; or when the doctor told me to write a will just before my lung surgery; or when I was told I had a rare cancer, I had faced death three times. Living through these three experiences and their aftermaths, I have learnt that no matter how bad things may seem, you need to accept your circumstances and look to move forward. Remember, good things also lay ahead of you, not just the bad. Since Layla was born, our family has expanded, as has Beyond Pain. It hasn't been all rosy though, not at all, but for me, accepting my circumstances and moving forward has been really important.

Yes, I have chronic pain; some have called it fibromyalgia, others have called it neuropathic pain and even phantom skin sensations. Ultimately it didn't matter what it's called; pain is pain, and I chose life. I chose to learn from my experiences, accept my situation and move forward with a purpose: a life beyond pain. My logo is *beyond pain* and I left a T-shirt with my logo hanging from the roof of Snowland Lodge in Phakding, Nepal.

Learn from your experiences, accept your situation and move forward with a purpose. Identify and use opportunities that are right in front of you. Choose a life beyond pain.

There is a way!

It is in the humble offering of my story that I hope you can make a difference to your life.

PART 2

THE UNDERSTANDING

INTRODUCTION

Why do we shake our hand wildly after we jam our fingers? Why do some people feel pain in the absence of injury? And why do we sometimes feel pain in a different place to the injured part? Pain is complex, but if we can understand it, then we can begin to conquer it.

If you have a better understanding of your pain and what is needed to manage it, you will feel more confident when dealing with it, no matter how hard it may seem. It will also lead you to become more proactive, instead of being fearful and reactive.

From personal experience, having a thorough understanding has allowed me to manage my pain with confidence. I no longer feel anxious about getting a flare-up of pain, rather, capable dealing with it.

In my clinic, a large part of my rehabilitation program is about education and understanding. My clients tell me how much more confident they feel in dealing with their pain because they know more about it.

Knowledge is power.

And the results don't lie.

I can help anyone who comes to my clinic with a willingness to learn and try something new.

This section uncovers the truths about pain, gives you an understanding of what pain is, and what strategies are most effective in conquering it.

PAIN: WHAT IS IT?

To address a problem, you first need to know what you are dealing with. Pain is no exception. Pain comes in many different forms and occurs for many different reasons – sometimes, for no obvious reason. Regardless of whether you have a nerve lesion, a bulging disc, fibromyalgia, a new injury, an old injury or no injury at all, the strategies covered in this book will help.

One of the biggest issues for people with pain is a lack of understanding of it. It follows logically then that, if you do understand pain, you can better manage it. Of course, you also need to have a helpful mindset, and if you add to that, relaxation techniques and properly-paced activities, it will make a world of difference.

Pain is complex. Pain is often described in vague terms such as: *an unpleasant sensory and emotional experience associated with actual or potential tissue damage.*

So what on earth does that actually mean?

It means that pain is more than just a simple physical sensation. Some feel the pain from an injury, while others feel the pain of a broken heart. Then there are those who have pain such as migraines where there is no injury, and amputees who have phantom pain in limbs they no longer possess.

So, yes, pain is complex.

ACUTE AND CHRONIC PAIN

When we talk about pain, we often talk about acute and chronic pain. Both can hurt just as much: pain is pain. The words *acute* and *chronic* refer to the length of time that pain persists. Here are simple definitions based on time:

- *Acute pain* is pain that lasts for up to three months.
- *Chronic pain* is pain that lasts for longer than three months, and is also known as persistent pain.

When you feel pain, your brain not only processes the pain messages from the injured body part, but it also processes your emotions, past experiences, and information from other senses such as touch, vision, hearing and temperature.

Let's see what this looks like.

Picture Nick. He works at an accounting firm and one day, he helps the office manager with a delivery of printer paper. As he bends over to lift a box of paper, he feels a sudden sharp stabbing pain and hears a cracking noise in his back. Nick immediately thinks that he must have a slipped disc because that was exactly what had happened to a mate of his who ended up being bedridden for six months. Nick begins to panic because he can't afford to be off work for six months, and just last week, he had calculated that he has only two weeks of sick leave. And if he doesn't get paid, how can he afford the deposit for the family holiday to Bali that he'd promised his wife and kids. The pain he feels is made much worse by his ensuing panic. The office manager looks over with great concern as Nick clutches his lower back.

Now picture Nick twenty minutes later. He is sitting in the tea room, having a cup of tea. He has taken some pain-killers, gently stretched out his back and walked around for a few minutes. The pain has reduced to a dull ache. Nick smiles to himself as he realises that it's not as bad as he first thought.

While Nick probably doesn't give it much thought, and gets on with his day as soon as he feels okay, his reaction and panic was caused not only by the initial sharp pain, but also by the cracking sound he heard, the look of concern on the office manager's face and knowledge of his friend who had suffered a back injury and had his whole life negatively affected. The physical pain was only one part of his pain experience. The rest was his brain adding all of its understandings and memories to the equation.

When you put all this into perspective, you can see why pain, whether it is acute or chronic, is more complicated than most people imagine – it is an experience unique to each person, and much more than a mere sensation. It is a complex body and brain response.

We have known this for thousands of years. The Greek philosopher and scientist, Aristotle, once said that, 'The treatment of the part should never be attempted without treatment of the whole. That is the error of our day, the separation of the body from the soul.' All those years ago, he understood, even though he was disregarded by his peers who all believed that if you had a pain in your leg, you needed to focus on the leg and nothing else.

PAIN MESSAGES

Even though pain messages from an injury are only one aspect of the pain experience, they are important and vital for survival. When we accidentally touch a hot stove, we feel a pain response and quickly pull our hand out of harm's way. Feeling pain helps us to learn to avoid harm. We wouldn't survive for long if we couldn't feel pain.

Pain messages are the body's way of letting us know that there is something amiss; it is like a personal alarm going off. Pain shouldn't be ignored, and most of us are good at responding to a pain message. If we have a headache or a sore neck, we take a painkiller. If we injure ourselves, we seek medical attention. The real problem occurs when the pain messages don't stop and our pain moves from acute to chronic – or from short-term to long-term.

TREATING ACUTE AND CHRONIC PAIN

Health practitioners are very good at treating acute pain. When a person goes to a doctor with pain, he or she is assessed, and perhaps sent for some tests and scans, and then a diagnosis is made. Effective treatment is provided and the pain usually goes away.

Even though we've all heard the phrase *see your doctor if pain persists*, health practitioners are not as good at treating chronic pain. Many try to treat it like acute pain – find the cause and then treat it.

The problem with chronic pain is that often there is no obvious cause, but undaunted, most doctors send patients for test after test to try and find a cause. If no cause can be found, these doctors often settle for a generalised label to describe the symptoms. Worse still, if a doctor can't find a label, the patient suffers while waiting for a diagnosis that might never come. Irrespective of whether a diagnosis is made, the patient's worry and frustration actually makes the pain worse.

Chronic pain should be treated like diabetes or asthma, both of which are currently, chronic conditions without cures. The best way to treat diabetes or asthma is to have an effective management plan. Diabetics and asthmatics don't focus on cures, but instead they focus on managing their conditions to live as normal a life as they can.

People with chronic pain need to do the same.

Sometimes, when the cause of the chronic pain can't be found, the pain itself can be dismissed or labelled as psychological, implying it is imaginary. Just because you can't see it, there is nothing imaginary about pain. The fact that you feel it – for whatever reason – means that it is real. Many people suffering chronic pain get frustrated when people tell them: 'you seem fine to me,' or even worse, 'if the doctors can't find anything wrong, it must be all in your head.'

This book explains why most chronic pain conditions can't be seen on scans and x-rays, and why it is common for chronic pain to exist in the absence of a definitive diagnosis. The reality is that irrespective of a diagnosis, you still need a sound understanding of the pain, which will lead to confidence, empowerment and a more helpful state of mind for you and the people trying to help you.

If you find a clinician who understands this, the results can be life changing.

THE HARDWARE AND SOFTWARE

Research shows that those who have a better understanding of their pain deal with it more successfully than those who don't. Understanding how your body works takes the mystery out of chronic pain. What follows is an overview of how pain works in your body. Some of this might surprise you.

THE NERVOUS SYSTEM

Just as the heart, arteries and veins are the hardware for circulation, the nervous system is the hardware for pain. The nervous system is made up of billions of nerve cells and is divided into two main parts: the central nervous system, which consists of the brain and spinal cord, and the peripheral nervous system, which consists of all the other nerves and nerve cells in the body.

The pain pathway involves both systems. The peripheral nervous system sends the pain messages, and in the central nervous system, the spinal cord relays the messages to the brain which processes the messages.

THE PERIPHERAL NERVOUS SYSTEM

The peripheral nervous system forms a dense network of nerves and nerve cells that constantly communicates with the central nervous system. When you have an injury, pain sensors are triggered and messages travel along the peripheral nervous system into your spinal cord and then up to your brain. Once your brain has processed these messages, your brain then sends instructions out through the spinal cord, to the peripheral nervous system, and onto your muscles and tissues to try to address the situation: your body's response.

THE SPINAL CORD

The spinal cord filters information that comes in from the body to go to the brain, just like a personal assistant filtering telephone calls to the boss. Your spinal cord only sends information to the brain that is important or information that has been requested by your brain. For example, can you feel your wrist watch? If you think about it, you can, but did you feel it ten minutes ago? Probably not. Until you thought about it and your brain requested information about your watch, your spinal cord was filtering out this information because it was not important.

THE BRAIN

The brain is the processing centre. Different areas of the brain help process different information. For example, there are sections of the brain that process thoughts, feelings, memories, and sensations such as touch, taste, movement, hearing, vision and speech. Because pain consists of both physical and emotional aspects, it is processed in several of these areas.

For a long time, health practitioners believed that the pathway from an injured site to the brain was simple: a single pathway takes messages from the injury to the spinal cord and then to the brain where the information is processed as pain.

Now we know it isn't that simple.

A lot of new ideas were explored after the world wars. There were many reports of soldiers with horrific injuries who hadn't felt any pain in the heat of battle. It wasn't until they were in safer territory that they felt pain. These soldiers weren't in shock – they reported none of the symptoms of cold, confusion or lack of focus – but their brains prioritised survival, and put the pain on hold.

Another thing puzzled scientists. Soldiers who had amputations reported feeling pain in limbs that were no longer there. These reports couldn't be explained by the long-held understanding of the simple pathway of pain.

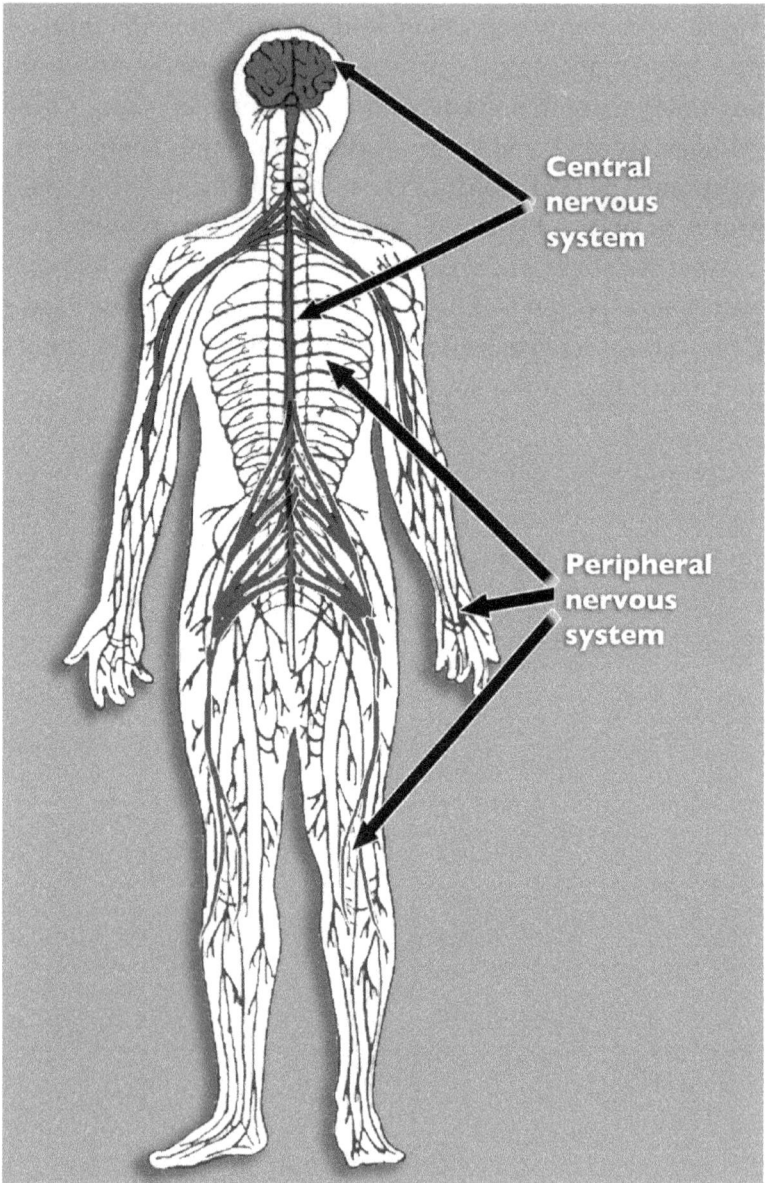

Central nervous system

Peripheral nervous system

The nervous system

THE NERVOUS SYSTEM IS LIKE A STREET MAP

As the figure below illustrates, an easy way to explain pain is to think of the nervous system as a street map. In this map:

- your nerves are the roads
- messages that run along the nerves are the traffic
- parts of your body (back, hands, legs etc.) are the outer suburbs
- your spinal cord is the inner suburbs
- your brain is the city centre.

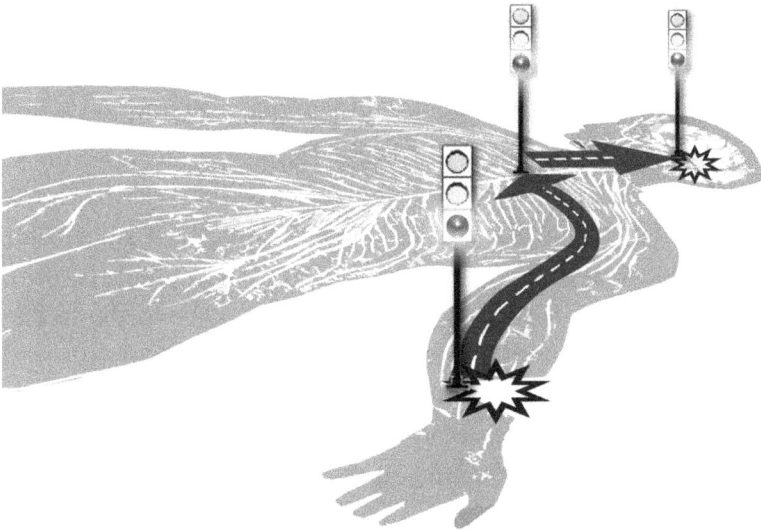

The nervous system is like a street map

To put it simply, the peripheral nervous system delivers messages from the body to the spinal cord, which then sends them to the brain; like traffic flowing from the outer suburbs (body) to the inner suburbs (the spinal cord) and then into the city (brain).

In the spinal cord, there are separate nerve highways for

pain, touch, movement, and temperature. When messages reach the spinal cord, they are sorted and directed into their respective highways. The pain messages go up the pain highway, temperature messages go up the temperature highway and so on.

These highways are connected by a network of smaller nerves (nerve cells), just like the network of backstreets that link road highways. As with road highways in peak hour, if a nerve highways' traffic backs up, messages can travel the smaller nerves and switch to a different nerve highway to get to the brain.

CONTROLLING THE FLOW OF PAIN TRAFFIC

Evolution has refined our response to pain so that it can best serve us. There are points along the main nerve highways that act like traffic lights. These block or allow messages to pass up the spinal cord, just like traffic lights controlling traffic flow on the roads. There is a reason for this system.In the heat of battle, soldiers don't feel the pain of an injury until they get to safety. In other words, in the heat of battle, the traffic lights on the pain highway turn red and don't allow the pain messages through. Traffic lights in the spinal cord are controlled by:

  · the volume of traffic on the highways
  · the brain
  · our thoughts and feelings.

Let's look at this more closely.

VOLUME OF TRAFFIC

Depending on the volume of traffic in the nervous system, the traffic lights on any particular highway will change from red to green. And, just like traffic flow on the roads during peak hour, the greater the traffic on a particular highway, the longer the lights stay green to let it through.

The amount of traffic required to turn the spinal cord lights from red to green is known as a *threshold*. Some highways have lower thresholds and require less traffic to turn the lights to green than other highways. For example, the touch and temperature highways have green lights most of the time because they have low thresholds. This is why we can feel a light touch or a slight temperature change. Normally, there isn't any traffic on the pain highway because its threshold is much higher. Its lights are usually red, which is why *normally*, we are mostly pain free. To put it very simply, people with chronic pain are likely to have more green lights on their pain highway.

When it comes to pain, every one is different. Some people will feel pain more quickly than others because these thresholds not only vary depending on the type of highway, but also vary from person to person.

THE BRAIN

These traffic lights are also controlled, to a degree, by the brain. If the brain wants more information, it sends messages to the spinal cord to turn the traffic lights on the relevant highway to green. Take the wrist watch example. If you are wearing a watch, you hardly notice it. If someone then mentions your watch, you immediately notice it and feel the sensation of wearing it. During this process, your brain selectively sends a message to the traffic lights on the touch highway to turn green and allow the messages about the watch to reach your brain.

Also, think back to the soldiers who didn't feel their shocking injuries in the heat of battle. If the brain perceives a situation to be life threatening, it will send messages to the spinal cord to turn all the lights on the pain highway to red so that it can concentrate on getting to safety. This is what we call the fight or flight response. Once out of danger, the brain sends messages to change the lights to green to assess the damage. This explains why the injured soldiers didn't feel any pain in the heat of battle, but felt it once they were safe.

When I was hit with the petrol bomb, I didn't feel any pain. I could see myself on fire, I could see my burning skin, but I couldn't feel any pain. It was a surreal situation. It wasn't until I got myself away from the fire to the relative safety of the bath, and when my brain knew that I was out of immediate danger, that the pain really kicked in.

As a less extreme example, think about the last time you tried to carry a hot plate. Your fingers and hands may have started to feel uncomfortably hot, but you managed to get the hot plate to the table before you really started feeling the pain. Here, your brain would have blocked pain messages until the task had been completed.

THOUGHTS AND EMOTIONS

One of the most important things to understand about pain is that thoughts and emotions can affect pain levels. When you feel positive, happy, calm or confident, your body produces endorphins – or *feel-good* hormones – which act as natural painkillers. Endorphins are very strong and can have pain-relieving effects that are similar to morphine but without the side effects.

Endorphins cause chemical reactions at the spinal cord which help turn the traffic lights on the pain highway to red, and stop or reduce the volume of messages reaching the brain. This explains why a lot of my clients say that they tend to feel less pain when they are playing with their children, out with friends or at the park with the grandkids.

Feeling low, angry or frustrated decreases the level of endorphins, and increases the level of the stress hormone, cortisol, both of which keep traffic lights green on the pain highway. As a result, people notice their aches and pains more when they feel anxious, angry or low. They may also feel more tension in their muscles or break out in a sweat as physical responses to their mood. Because of this, we really need to be aware of how our thoughts and emotions affect our pain.

PUTTING IT TOGETHER

Imagine you jam your fingers in a drawer. Pain messages from your hand travel to the spinal cord through the peripheral nervous system. Once these messages reach the spinal cord, they are filtered into the pain highway, and the sudden volume of traffic turns the traffic lights on the pain highway to green, and the messages travel up to the brain.

When your brain processes these messages, it recognises that they have come from your fingers, and obtains information from other senses, such as the reddened skin you can see, the jamming sound you heard and the rapid swelling of your fingers that you felt. Your brain then mixes all of these with your thoughts, emotions and memories of any past injuries to create a pain *experience*. The brain then sends messages to the traffic lights on the pain highway to keep them green to learn more about the pain.

Once the initial stages of the injury have passed, fewer pain messages are sent to the spinal cord. There may be enough to keep some of the traffic lights green, but this time, because there are fewer messages, it is processed as just an ache. As days pass, your fingers continue to improve, pain messages stop, traffic lights turn to red on the pain highway, and there are no more pain messages travelling to your brain. As a result, your brain does not ask for more information. Everything goes back to normal.

Another interesting response can occur. Earlier, we talked about messages changing highways when there's congestion. If you jam your fingers and the pain highway becomes flooded with pain messages, some of the connecting nerve cells become activated. Some of the pain messages take these backstreets and switch to less congested highways, such as the temperature or touch highways. As a result, your pain may feel like a burning pain or a sharp pain. These inter-linking highways and backstreets show that pain is certainly not as simple as it might first appear.

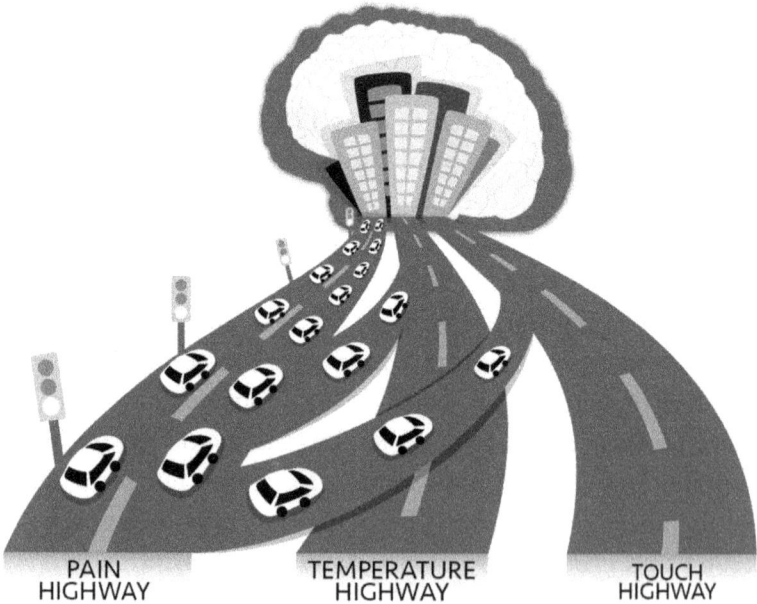

PAIN HIGHWAY   TEMPERATURE HIGHWAY   TOUCH HIGHWAY

The Spinal Cord: When there is congestion, pain messages use less congested nerve highways to get to the brain, just like traffic on our roads using alternative routes during peak hour traffic.

THE SENSITIVE NERVOUS SYSTEM

People who suffer from chronic pain often have a nervous system that is more sensitive to pain. This sensitivity can happen after an injury or illness, or even just over time. While researchers don't know *why* it happens, they are learning more about *how* it happens. When there is a constant flow of messages over a long period of time, changes occur in the make-up of the nervous system causing the normal pain threshold to drop – making the nervous system more sensitive to pain. Sometimes this new sensitivity is confined to the site of the damage or injury, but it can spread to other areas. Scans and x-rays can't show a sensitive nervous system, and often patients visit many doctors to find a cause for their chronic pain without success before they are finally told that the sensitive nervous system is the cause.

CENTRAL SENSITISATION

If the traffic lights on the pain highway stay green for a long time, as happens with sufferers of chronic pain, a steady flow of messages reaches the brain. The brain wants to know more and sends signals to the spinal cord to keep the lights green. The traffic then builds up rapidly. The cycle continues and the sufferer constantly feels pain. As the volume of traffic builds up, the smaller network of backstreets is activated and pain messages cut through. If this continues, over time certain changes occur:

- the traffic lights on the pain highway turn green more quickly, even with fewer pain messages (threshold drops)
- the traffic lights stay green for longer
- the backstreets remain active and open, even when there is little traffic.

When people say that changes in the weather affect their pain, they are not lying. Think of your old uncle who can predict a change in the weather because his hip plays up. The weather doesn't *cause* the pain, but there *is* a pain response. What happens is that temperature messages have travelled along the temperature highway, but some have taken the backstreets and then switched to the pain highway, even though the temperature highway is not over-loaded. This backstreet jumping mixes up the sensations.

All these changes are collectively known as *central sensitisation*. Even though it sounds like a good name for a train station, it simply means that your spinal cord is more sensitive to pain than normal.

This explains the phenomenon of phantom pain. When amputees report feeling pain in a part of the body that has been removed, it's because the amputation have caused the traffic lights on the pain highway to remain on green for a lengthy period of time, causing the spinal cord to become sensitised.

DESENSITISING THE NERVOUS SYSTEM

When you jam your fingers, you instinctively shake your hand vigorously, rub your fingers, and maybe even blow onto it. So why do we do this? It is actually a primal body and brain response to counteract the pain messages. It helps reduce the pain.

Here's how.

When pain messages reach the brain, it calls for more information about the pain. The brain does this by keeping the traffic lights on the pain highway green. The brain seeks as much information as possible to be able to respond and protect the body. The more pain information the brain receives, the more it hurts.

To counter this, we instinctively try to take the brain's

attention away from the pain by giving it other signals to process. By shaking your hand, rubbing your fingers or blowing onto them, you are increasing traffic on the movement, touch and temperature highways, and increasing the number of other messages for your brain to process. As a consequence, your brain is distracted from the pain and sends fewer messages to the spinal cord wanting to know about the jammed-finger pain. With a decrease in messages from the brain, some lights turn back to red on the pain highway.

It's a bit like when there is major congestion on one of our road highways. All the traffic-reporting helicopters hover over this highway, reporting back to the newsroom. However, if the helicopters get information that the other highways are getting congested too, some will go and investigate. Therefore the newsroom's attention isn't solely on the first highway.

For the same reasons, heat and ice are used regularly with great effect in the treatment of chronic pain. Not only do they act as a therapeutic aid, but they also act as a distraction by using the temperature highway. The more information the brain has to process, the less time it has to focus on pain.

Shaking your hand is an effective means to distract your brain, even when you are dealing with chronic pain. But if you have chronic pain in your back, you can't simply shake it. What you can do is start stretching and exercising, and using your back. Total rest is not the solution for chronic pain.

Because people with chronic pain often have more than one painful area, the best treatment for most chronic pain conditions is to increase activity on the other highways but gradually building up activity levels, and by using strategies such as self-massage (touch) and heat/ice (temperature), so that the brain has a variety of information to process – not just pain.

Activity has many benefits. Activity gets the blood flooding to the damaged tissue; it increases the release of endorphins (the body's natural painkillers), which help turn the traffic lights to red on the pain highway. This, with other strategies like heat, ice, self-massage and relaxation techniques, can desensitise the nervous system and allow you to take control of your pain.

While you shouldn't ignore pain messages, if you have chronic pain and you are returning to activity, some discomfort is normal. This discomfort can be due to scar tissue, the skin over the affected area being oversensitive, or you might have tight muscles and ligaments. It may simply be that some movement messages have jumped across to the pain highway. You also might get an initial increase in pain because you are anxious about doing anything that might aggravate your injury, releasing chemicals that keep some of the lights on the pain highway green. But if you continue to be active, over time, you won't notice your pain as much. This is because activity helps not only to distract the brain, but also improves the health of your ligaments, strength and flexibility of your muscles and keeps your joints naturally lubricated.

A video explaining how pain works in your body can be viewed for free by scanning the QR code or visiting www.beyondpain.com.au and navigating to the 'Downloads' page.

MAPPING THE PAIN

To make you more aware of your body, your brain develops a map based on your activity levels. The more active you are, the more information your brain receives to develop the map. Some body parts, such as your hands and your mouth, are mapped with great accuracy because you use these parts more frequently.

When you are in pain, you can usually say exactly where your pain is, thanks to your body map. But when you have chronic pain, you are generally less active and your body map becomes blurred. This is why most people with chronic pain find it difficult to pin-point the exact location of their pain.

When you become active again, your body map is updated, and the blurring generally lessens. This is why if you have a back injury, and rest, the pain feels as if it is all over your back. Start being active and the pain becomes more localised to a particular area of your back: your brain has re-mapped your back and can identify with greater accuracy where the pain actually is.

Pain specialists call this ability to map and re-map the body *neuroplasticity*. It just means that you can change and mould your body map, depending on what you do, just like plastic. Activity really can help in many ways.

While being active is important, take care not to fall into the trap of overdoing things. Don't do what I did and compete in a triathlon without any preparation and training. Start by doing an amount of activity that is *comfortable* and *manageable*, and gradually build it up. Also be aware of delays in pain responses. Sometimes because your body's natural painkillers are released during activity, you may not notice the pain as much.

Be a little conservative.

THE VICIOUS CYCLE

The chronic pain vicious cycle is common. Without even realising, people get themselves into a cycle where they focus on their pain, stop talking to their family or friends, stop working or exercising and stop having a good quality of life. As a result, their pain worsens, and their life becomes all about the pain. This chapter explains how that cycle happens, and more importantly, explains how you can avoid it, or, get out of it if you find yourself caught in it.

GETTING CAUGHT UP IN THE CYCLE

Your thoughts and feelings affect your level of pain. This is a fact. When you are in pain, having unhelpful thoughts will work against you. But having helpful thoughts will lead to you feeling better and an increase in the production of feel-good hormones. Further, feeling good makes you less likely to avoid activity.

We know that avoiding or significantly reducing activity causes muscles to weaken, ligaments to tighten and joints to stiffen. When your body is like this, you feel even worse. Most people in pain get caught up in this cycle. The really negative thing about this cycle is that you end up focusing more on your symptoms, and the more you focus on how bad you feel, the worse you *will* feel.

When your body is out of condition and you try to do something like gardening or shopping, you will really feel it. And because you feel pain with even a little bit of activity, in most cases, you try and avoid doing things altogether. This is the vicious cycle, and in a diagram, it looks like this:

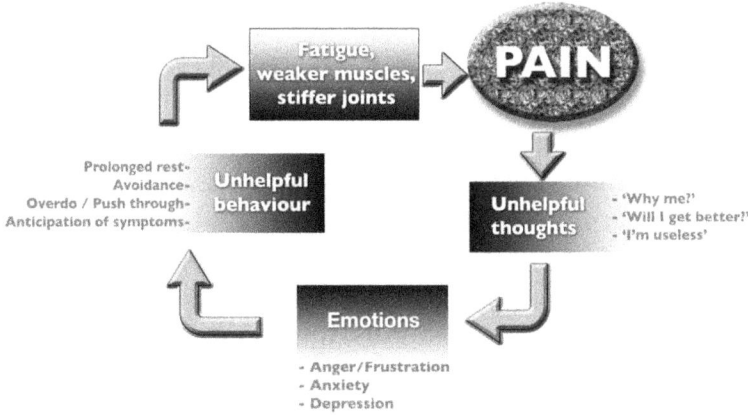

The vicious cycle

It doesn't stop there. This vicious cycle can lead to secondary problems and other symptoms such as weight gain, poor sleep and a lack of mobility. You focus more on your symptoms, and end up doing only the things you have to do, like working, cleaning and shopping. The things that you may enjoy doing – socialising and pursuing hobbies – can be relegated to the bottom of your priority list. Unfortunately some people don't understand that doing the things you enjoy actually helps to release your body's natural painkillers. They are, therefore, just as important as the things you have to do.

Remember, your pain is more than just physical symptoms. When you are caught in this vicious cycle, all aspects of your life can be affected.

WORK, FINANCIAL AND SOCIAL FACTORS

Sometimes people with chronic pain stop working. You may be one of those people. It may be just too painful to continue, or you may think that working will cause further pain. You might be motivated to work, but simply feel that you can't.

Returning to work with chronic pain isn't easy, but it is important.

Research shows that the longer you are off work, the worse your health and pain become. Not only that, but the longer you don't work, the less likely you are ever to return to work. Don't forget that work isn't just about money. It gets you out of the house, it makes you feel valued, it gives you a routine, it has a social element, and at the end of the day, it helps you to sleep better because it has drained your energy.

Some people think that if they can't perform like they used to, they would rather not be at work at all. This all-or-nothing attitude can prevent people from returning to work. The problem is that sometimes we don't even realise that we think this way. This certainly happened to me when I was recovering from my burns. I was frustrated that people around me had to help me in one way or another, and sub-consciously, I think I just wanted to get better first before I thought about work so that I didn't have to rely on anyone. But now I realise how beneficial getting back to work was for my recovery. Returning to work is a part of returning to life. I now appreciate the key role it played in my reha-bilitation.

Work is not something that should happen *after* your rehabilitation. Work is a *part* of your rehabilitation.

The financial cost of not working also needs to be con-sidered. It may mean that your quality of life diminishes. Bills mount up and benefit payments are never the same as your wage. Your social life may suffer because you can't afford to go out, or you might worry that your friends are sick of hearing about your pain at a time when you have little else to talk about in your life. For me, it really hit home when the monthly rent was due, the electricity bill landed on our dining table, and when my mobile phone credit ran out. And I was only responsible for myself – I wasn't supporting a family. It didn't feel good to scrape through month-by-month, and say no to my friends when they asked me out because I couldn't afford it. In so many ways, pain can really diminish your self-worth.

Being off work often also affects sleep and concentration. When you are not working, your mental and physical energy remains in your body and at night you feel restless and unable to sleep properly. This can directly affect your concentration and focus during the day. If you haven't been able to work for a long period of time, but you are keen to get back, it's never too late. Time after time, clients tell me that they can't work, or that doctors have told them they can't work, and they've almost given up hope. But I can assure you that almost every client who has wanted to return to work has done so.

FAMILY

If you are unable to work, your family may also be affected. If you are a parent, you may not be able to support your children in the same manner as before, which may lead to feelings of frustration and depression. You may become angry at yourself and lash out at your family. You may even feel guilty and isolate yourself from your family. This is what pain can do to a person.

There were several times when this happened to me. I remember a time when I was in hospital after my skin graft and I snapped at my parents when all they wanted to do was help. Even now, I remember my feelings of frustration and helplessness. At that moment, I just wanted to be left alone. But I was surprised by my own outburst; this wasn't the real me.

Sometimes your family might insist that you rest without knowing that it is not beneficial for you to do so. They may even do your share of the housework thinking that they are being helpful. But they may not know that inactivity makes things worse, or that you may feel bad about not pulling your weight. Alternatively, they might get frustrated at you for not helping. All of this adds to the pain.

DOING THE ROUNDS

People will do anything and pay almost anything to find relief from pain. They will undergo tests and scans, take medications, and seek second, third and fourth opinions from a range of doctors and therapists. Most treatments are successful in treating acute pain, but generally, they only offer temporary relief from chronic pain. The problem with chronic pain is that, in most cases, there is often no identifiable cause. A lot of time and money is spent looking for a cure, only for the pain to continue and often worsen. You may begin to lose hope and the chronic pain may seem as if it has total control of your life, further adding to your pain experience. No wonder people get confused and lose their way. See what this looks like in a diagram:

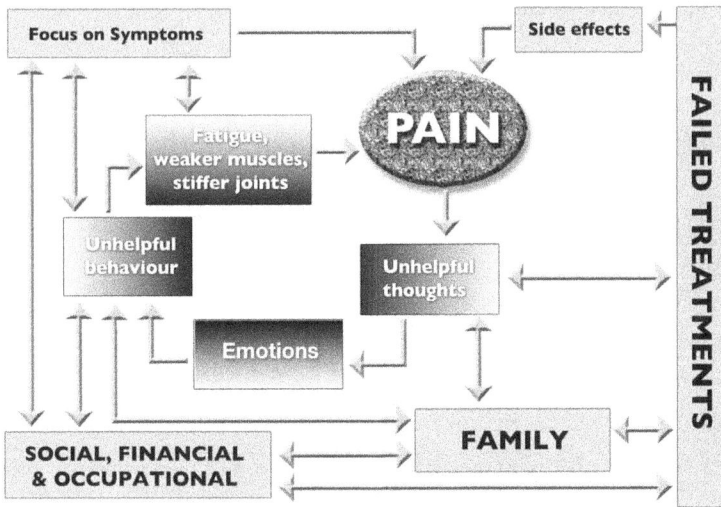

The factors that can affect the vicious cycle

You may not have understood this cycle until now, and simply blamed your pain for the situation you find yourself in. When this tumultuous cycle persists, you start to anticipate pain and other symptoms. You may start to avoid more and more activities and not commit to any social functions because you just don't know if you will be up to it. People with chronic pain can feel as if their fight is futile and that the pain has defeated them. A recent study in the United Kingdom of 133 people with chronic pain, found that the higher the feelings of mental defeat, the worse the reported pain, depression and perceived disability. It is important to recognise and change this. You may feel overwhelmed by all of this, but keep reading. You will gain the knowledge and the skills to help you identify and make changes that will turn things around, just like I did.

THE ULTIMATE GOAL

We all strive to achieve different things, but sometimes we lose sight of the ultimate goal: getting your life back. People become so busy being proactive in their search for a cure for chronic pain that they don't realise the best treatment comes when they look to the future and identify their goals and aspirations, *despite* the pain.

When your focus shifts away from the pain, and back onto improving your lifestyle, a happier lifestyle will result, which will inevitably lead to less pain. Your goals should include both the things you *need* to do and enjoyable things you *want* to do. *Accept* that your pain may be here to stay and *believe* in your ability to live a rewarding active life. Pain originates from your body – you have control of your body – and, therefore, you can take control of your pain. While in most cases there may not be a cure for it, pain can only take control of your life if you let it. Your thinking has to change from:

My pain is my life

to

My pain is a part of my life that I will manage.

THE NEVER-ENDING REFERRALS

Health practitioners are in the business because they genuinely want to help people. If someone comes into a doctor's surgery with pain, the doctor genuinely wants to help them to get better by first trying to identify the cause. The problem for people with chronic pain is that often there is no diagnosis or identifiable cause for what they are feeling.

Most doctors follow a traditional medical model in their practices: identify the symptoms, find and diagnose the cause, then treat it. People with chronic pain can often spend months going from specialist to specialist trying to find a cause before commencing any treatment. Some people think that visiting specialists is being proactive, but they don't realise that, despite all these appointments, they aren't actually being treated for their pain.

I mostly see patients who have done the rounds of the medical profession before coming to me. You may be able to relate to this. This chapter explores why this happens, and shows you that there is another way.

DOCTOR HOPPING

The pursuit of a diagnosis for acute pain conditions is necessary. Identifying a discernible cause of pain, such as a torn ligament or a bone fracture, is important to the treatment of the condition. In terms of diagnosis, many in the healthcare professions don't distinguish between acute and chronic pain. This sends you on a hunt for a diagnosis and the consequential specialist hopping.

It all starts when your doctor sends you for an ultrasound to identify the cause of, say, your sore foot. You then have a follow-up appointment with your doctor who tells you that they can't really see anything, but that maybe you should get an x-ray. You go for the x-ray, but the x-ray doctor says that the images don't show any cause for your pain. They suggest you see an orthopaedic surgeon. You wait weeks for the appointment and see the surgeon who sends you for an MRI. A couple of weeks later, you see the surgeon again for the MRI results. They tell you that you have some osteoarthritis in your joints. The surgeon also says that there's nothing much they can do about it and sends you back to your doctor.

'Take these painkillers,' your doctor says, and hands you a script.

After a while, the painkillers stop working, so you ring your doctor and ask what else can be done because you are too young to be hobbling around like an invalid.

'Maybe a rheumatologist,' they suggest.

Off to the rheumatologist you go with all your scans and reports in one hand and the referral in the other. They look through everything and decides to inject you with cortisone which brings relief for a couple of months. When it starts hurting again, you go back and get another shot. A couple of years drift by with regular injections and the my-foot-feels-good and now-it-hurts cycle repeating itself like ground-hog day. Finally, the cortisone stops working and the rheumatologist suggest you see another specialist. You go back to your doctor for yet another referral.

No wonder the painting *The Scream* by Edvard Munch comes to mind for most with chronic pain. By the time you go to a pain management clinic, you may have seen at least half a dozen doctors and specialists, spent a lot of time and money, but only to end up with the same outcome: no diagnosis, no long-term benefits from treatment, and still, the same chronic pain.

INTERNET DIAGNOSIS

With the internet being such a prominent part of our lives, it's only natural that you might search for answers online. There are some very helpful sites that are run by reputable organisations and offer useful information about chronic pain. But there seems to be many more sites that aren't as helpful. Some of these unhelpful sites suggest radical treatments and potentially dangerous quick fixes, while others paint a very bleak picture of your situation. In desperation, some people take on suggestions given on these sites with dire consequences.

Remember, most of these sites and forums are frequented by people who aren't health professionals and who haven't successfully managed their pain. These people usually only talk about their negative experiences, and this might leave you in a more fearful or worried state. You need to keep in mind that the people who are successfully managing their pain are busy living their lives, not discussing their issues on the internet. So while getting appropriate information from trustworthy sites on the internet may help, be mindful about entering uninformed websites and forums.

LOSING FOCUS OF THE ULTIMATE GOAL

You can begin to feel like a silver ball in a pinball machine. You get flicked from doctor to doctor, test to test, specialist to specialist. Of course, your doctor has the best of intentions; they just want to help you. But there is an emotional cost to you – the ongoing frustrations and disappointment, and the uncertainty of not having a diagnosis. There is also often a considerable financial cost to you and society. Billions of dollars are spent each year in Australia on the unsuccessful diagnosis and treatment of chronic pain conditions.

The problem with searching for a diagnosis for chronic pain is that often there isn't one. People can doctor-hop for years and still be none the wiser, and still in pain.

Want to hear a different plan of attack? I strongly believe that you would be better off focusing your energy into *managing the pain*, rather than seeking the reason for it, or at least doing both.

The very act of doctor hopping can, I feel, distract you from the ultimate goal.

So what is the goal?

If you ask people with chronic pain, most will say, 'to get rid of the pain.'

But even if a magic pain-fairy waved a wand and made the pain disappear, you would still have to establish new work and daily routines, re-establish your social life, re-introduce activity, and learn to see yourself in a different light.

So while the goal is to be free of the pain, what everyone really wants – in the big picture – is get back to having a happy life.

What if you aim for the happy life first, rather than trying to find a cure for your pain?

Think of it like this. You're all dressed up to go to a fabulous party on a yacht that is leaving at 8 pm. You've selected the perfect outfit and you look a million dollars. In the limo on the way there with all your friends, one of them spills a glass of champagne down the front of your outfit. You are left with two choices: either clean up what you can and continue while accepting that there is a blemish on your outfit, or you get out of the limo and catch a cab home. The reality is that, if you were to go out on the yacht, you would probably have too much fun to notice you even have a blemish.

Pain management is a bit like the party dilemma. If attending the party is your ultimate goal, choosing to accept the blemish on your outfit is what you have to do to get there and enjoy yourself. If living a happy lifestyle is your ultimate goal, then accepting your pain and making the decision to do the most helpful things to achieve your goal is what you have to do. And like the blemish, when you start to enjoy life again, you will notice your pain less.

LEARNED HELPLESSNESS

Understandably, there are a lot of people with chronic pain who look for cures. Following the traditional medical model, doctors start the search and specialists continue it. The patient is then supposed to do their bit by getting better.

But this model does not work with chronic pain.

That doesn't stop the health practitioners. In their diligence, they can continue to give you temporary relief, even if the treatment offers you no lasting benefits. An example of this is a physiotherapist who can massage someone with chronic back pain and make them feel better for a couple of hours or even a couple of days. They do this because they feel like they are helping by giving some relief, figuring that it's better than nothing. The problem is that this temporary relief doesn't help in the long run. It is costly and repetitive and offers no ultimate solutions.

The clinician's attempts to help can also give false hope. If the doctor won't give up until they find a cure, then that must mean there is a cure to be found.

Unfortunately, some people with chronic pain become

reliant on regular treatments that only offer short-term relief, and even begin to plan their lives around them: *I can't go on holiday because I can't miss my physio appointment.* Clinically, this is called *learned helplessness.* It's common for people to insist on continuing to receive a treatment, even after their clinician has told them it's not helping. This may be you.

If you enjoy a good massage, there is nothing wrong with having one, but it is not the answer for managing chronic pain in the longer term. It should be a treat, not a treatment.

That's not to say that traditional therapies don't have a place in chronic pain management. When you are experiencing a flare-up of pain, having one or two sessions of physiotherapy or acupuncture, or temporarily using medication might be the right thing for you. But don't fall into the trap of becoming reliant on these or other such treatments for chronic pain flare-ups.

The true long-term solution lies in a different approach.

WHAT THE RESEARCH TELLS US

Many doctors and health professionals know a lot about acute pain, but not necessarily a lot about chronic pain. It makes sense – you hurt yourself, you go to your doctor. Remember our definition for chronic pain – it is pain that has persisted for more than three months. And remember our point that, because health practitioners treat acute pain all the time, they often treat chronic pain in the same way.

There has been a lot of research done into which treatments work for chronic pain. Recent research into the way that doctors treat chronic lower back pain found that most doctors treat it according to their own beliefs. One might use acupuncture, while another might prescribe medication and rest. The research found a lack of consensus among doctors on the most appropriate treatment. The approach was generally based on intervention rather than management. In other words, doctors tried to fix the problem rather than manage it. While this may be fine for people who've strained a back muscle or slept funny and woken up with a crick in their neck, it is not helpful to people with chronic pain.

Such approach doesn't provide a long-term solution. The best long-term solution is in learning to manage the pain.

A study in the United Kingdom looked at the beliefs that doctors had about chronic pain. The study showed that most doctors recommend that their patients avoid activity to avoid pain. But this lack of understanding will actually increase their patients' pain levels.

So why don't most doctors know the best ways to treat chronic pain?

When I studied physiotherapy, chronic pain management wasn't mentioned at all. I graduated in 2000. Universities have begun to incorporate some sessions on chronic pain management into their course curriculums, but more needs to be done for things to change.

It is estimated that one in five people suffer from chronic pain – that's 20 per cent of the population. To put this in perspective, more people suffer from chronic pain than asthma and diabetes combined. And depending on which website you visit or research paper you read, estimates are that chronic pain costs Australia over $30 billion and over 10 million absent days each year. Around the world, the total cost is estimated to exceed US$300 billion annually. We have to ask ourselves why *all* health professionals aren't learning how to best treat it.

You'd also hope it would be in the interest of governments to embrace the most successful treatments for chronic pain; it could save billions.

THE OVERACTIVITY–UNDERACTIVITY ROLLERCOASTER

An unhelpful pattern that people with chronic pain get into is trying to do too much and then crashing down with more pain. You might relate to this. This chapter explains that there is a better way: gradually building up activity levels, or breaking up activities into manageable components.

RECOGNISING THE ROLLERCOASTER

Throughout our lives, there will be times when we overdo things. In today's hectic lifestyle, essential everyday activities such as shopping, cleaning, and cooking are demanding to everyone – not just people with chronic pain. These day-to-day activities become even more demanding when we overdo things to meet deadlines. We do this knowing that there is a holiday, a promotion, a bonus, or just a rest at the end of the hard work. It is a choice we make.

Unfortunately with chronic pain, there is no choice. Just completing everyday activities feels like hard work. When it feels this way, we are not inclined to take on extra demands – particularly when there is no end to the hardship in sight. You may feel like you are using all your strength and willpower just to get the basic necessities in life completed. You may have nothing left for more enjoyable activities. It's common for you to feel burnt out, disheartened and sick of the struggle. It may feel like the pain is in control of your life; it is your own private dictator.

My clients generally say that, over time, the number of good (or not so bad) days diminishes. Unfortunately, when trying to deal with their pain, sufferers can inadvertently get into some unhelpful patterns.

You might be familiar with some of these most common patterns where you:

- try to get a job done in one go, and then suffer the consequences
- try to push through your pain, and carry on until the pain becomes so unbearable that you must stop
- avoid activities that carry a risk of even the slightest increase in pain
- find it difficult to break up activities and want to complete things all in one go because that's how you've always done things
- become over-cautious about doing things because you worry that a sudden movement may cause severe pain or damage
- get others to do things that you once did yourself, instead of doing what you can and getting others to help
- prioritise day-to-day things and meet other people's needs rather than doing the things you enjoy.

Getting caught in these behaviours is like being on a rollercoaster. On better days, you tend to do basic chores like shopping, cleaning and mowing the lawn because you don't know when a really bad day is around the corner. You cram in all the jobs that have to be done, and despite increases in pain, you use willpower and perseverance to push on. That's the climb part of the rollercoaster ride.

At a certain point, the pain becomes too much and you

are overcome with exhaustion and despair, leaving you feeling run down, defeated and frustrated. That is when you free-fall down the rollercoaster.

To cope, you may take painkillers to try to get some relief. Initially, it may take only a couple of hours to recover. But every time you overdo things, your body becomes stiffer and you feel an increase in your pain sooner. And it takes longer to recover.

Before long, the same task becomes more and more difficult; your stamina and endurance lessens, and the pain worsens. You may become angry, develop unhelpful behaviours and your body becomes weaker and stiffer. Ironically, people who attempt too much, end up in the same place as people who didn't do much in the first place. Both end up losing condition. Their muscles weaken and joints tighten, and in that state, they don't feel like doing much at all.

Regularly pushing through the pain actually does more harm than good. It causes changes in the nervous system that result in a build-up of the pain intensity and reduces the pain threshold, meaning that over time you feel more pain and the pain comes on sooner.

The flow-on effect is an increase in rest periods. Before, it might have taken you days to recover, but now it takes weeks. You begin to anticipate the pain and other symptoms. You let your pain be the guide as to how much you can do because your main focus is always to ease the pain. That is why, over time, the number of good days become fewer.

One of my clients, a 50-year-old man called Jim, had arthritis in his knees. His doctor had advised him to do short walks to increase the strength and stability of his knees, but Jim thought that if he did half as many longer walks, it would amount to the same thing. The longer walks hurt, but Jim thought it must be doing him some good. Jim increased the distance he walked, and not only that, he thought that if he went faster, there would be even greater benefit. Four days after he began his new long-walk routine, Jim woke up with really sore knees that were too sore for him to get up. He spent the next week lying on the couch, frustrated. While he was recuperating, he could see his beloved lawn out the window and it was looking untidy. When he began to feel better, the lawn was his first priority. He pushed his old lawn mower around his big backyard, just wanting to get the job done. He pushed through his pain, but afterwards, he took even longer to recover. He couldn't believe how much of a struggle a simple task like mowing had become. His anger and frustration deepened as he lay on the couch with his knees hurting more than ever. When his frustration and anger diminished, Jim started to worry instead; he couldn't see any light at the end of the tunnel.

This is the point most of my clients are at when they first come to me.

People often use pain as a guide to avoid further damage and injury because instinctively, pain is perceived as a threat. While this is useful in acute pain where you need to listen to your pain – a sprained ankle, a burn or a broken arm – it is not so helpful for chronic pain where the pain is more inconsistent. It is common for people to report more pain when they are less active, and less pain on days they have been more active. For many, this is difficult to understand.

If you use your pain levels as a guide, you can find your life really disrupted. If, on the other hand, you acknowledge your chronic pain and plan your life sensibly around it, you can live a rich and fulfilling life, despite the pain.

The key word here is *manageable*.

If a person does a manageable amount of activity that sits within their capability and comfort levels, or even slightly pushes their boundaries, they will be able to build on that and improve.

If a person overdoes things, they are not allowing their bodies to gently adapt to changes, and are constantly putting their bodies under stress and fatigue.

The phrase *no pain, no gain* does not apply to acute and chronic pain. *Know your pain to gain* better fits the pain sufferer.

What also doesn't work is the *no movement, no pain, no worries* lifestyle that some people follow. When people try to avoid aggravating their pain by being over-cautious, they are, in fact, letting their pain decide what they can and can't do.

Overactivity-underactivity Rollercoaster

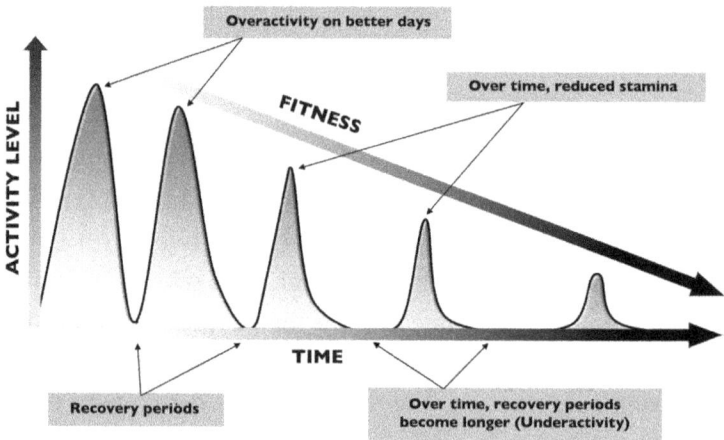

The overactivity-underactivity rollercoaster – the peaks represent high levels of activity, followed by less activity when we feel exhausted. Over time, we do less, rest more, and our fitness declines

ADVANTAGES AND DISADVANTAGES OF THE ROLLERCOASTER

Why do people get on the overactivity–underactivity rollercoaster if it's so detrimental? People, by nature, like to get things done. We have to-do lists and check lists to keep us on track. When people with chronic pain have a better day, they want to use it to their best advantage. And who can blame them?

Advantages	Disadvantages
• You get the job done.	• There is no consistency in what you do.
• You feel as though you achieved something.	• You often have to rest and recover, even when you haven't done a lot.
• You force yourself to do the important things.	• You can no longer plan because you need to wait and see how your pain is.
• You might have others offer to help you in your activity and so you spend more time with people.	• Your life starts to revolve around your pain.
• Being able to do things on the better days stops you from feeling like a failure.	• You get more pain before and after an activity, your rest periods become longer and you become tired more quickly.
• Pushing yourself to stay at work means there is food on the table. It also means you are useful.	• You feel as though you have to rush and do as much as possible before the pain gets unbearable.

• You contribute to your family in any way you are able to.

• Resting too much makes you feel tired, sluggish and bored. Your fitness suffers.

• You feel stressed, anxious, depressed, angry and frustrated.

• You wonder why you bother doing it in the first place if you end up with more pain.

• You feel weak and stiff.

• Life has become all work, and no play.

The advantages of the rollercoaster are definitely short-term. If you are in this pattern, the sooner you can recognise it and see that, in the long-term, it will not be helpful, the sooner you will be able to change your unhelpful habits to more helpful ones.

No matter how bad the habit, you can always change it. Once you are able to do this, you will be in a better position to establish a routine that incorporates work, rest and play.

The people who find it most difficult to break out of this pattern are those who strongly believe that they have *survived* by using the overactivity–underactivity roller-coaster. That may well be the case, but it doesn't need to be so hard.

Almost every person who is not successful in managing their pain falls into one of three categories: underac-tive, overactive, or a bad mixture of both. Read the true examples below to see if you can personally relate to any of the patterns.

THE UNDERACTIVE MAN

Former sales assistant, 26-year-old Michael, loved the outdoors and enjoyed playing football and hiking. His chronic pain is the result of a work injury four years ago when he tried to lift a new microwave oven off a shelf to show to a customer. Later, he told everyone that this one moment ruined his back forever. From that time on, he has been fearful of lifting anything heavy. A specialist told him that he needs to be careful with his back because his spine has a degenerative disease and that he may end up in a wheelchair if he isn't careful. Michael has physiotherapy twice a week, which includes a daily home exercise program. But he never did the home exercises because he was scared his back would *break* and he would end up in a wheelchair.

Now, every time he tries to do anything – even something as easy as standing up from his armchair – he feels back pain. Gone are the days of playing football and hiking. He hasn't done any of that since the initial incident. Michael has also stopped going out and socialising with friends. He says that, because his pain is unpredictable, he doesn't want to take the risk of being a party-pooper. Most of the time, Michael sits inactive at home thinking bitterly about the life he used to have and all the things he has lost. He says his life is ruined.

THE OVERACTIVE MUM

Sophia is a 44-year-old full-time cleaner who lives with her husband and three teenage daughters. She has aches and pains all over her body, but begins work at 7 o'clock each morning. After working an eight-hour day, she picks up her daughters from school, and then cooks dinner and helps her children with their homework. After dinner, she cleans up and makes the school lunches for the next day. By the time Sophia sits down for a cuppa, it's often well past 10 pm. During the weekend, she tries to clean the house, but she also has to run errands for her elderly parents. Because of her chronic pain – which a series of doctors has so far failed to diagnose – she has taken eight weeks of sick leave in the last year. She feels guilty at not pulling her weight both at work and at home. She has always been a get-on-with-the-job kind of person, but now she is slower and feels depressed most of the time.

THE OVERACTIVE AND UNDERACTIVE ROLLERCOASTER MAN

At 53, Bill has ongoing knee pain from a work accident three years ago. He varies his activity depending on how he feels. Some days he goes to work for a few hours, returns home and washes his car or finishes the list of jobs that his wife has stuck to the fridge. Bill likes to get everything done, and each day, he has to take a high dose of medication to allow him to keep going. Over time, Bill has realised that, although he has consistently tried to get everything done on the better days, he can no longer maintain such a high level of activity. When he crashes after doing too much, it takes him longer to recover, even if he tries to rest. He has also noticed that he sleeps for much longer than was used to. Bill has cut back his hours of work and now he only works part-time. He varies his start and finish times depending on how he feels each day. Bill can't understand why he is getting worse. He tries to soldier on regardless, but tends to crash and increasingly feels low and frustrated. Bill tries to fit in even more things on his better days to make up for what he can't do on the ever-increasing number of bad days.

GETTING IT RIGHT

What if you were able to get off the roller coaster? It is possible if you begin with a comfortable starting point for your exercises and activities, and build on them weekly. Gradually pick up the pace of the activity and monitor your progress. Stick to your manageable plan irrespective of your pain or how good you feel – your pain will then, not guide you. It's all in the pacing.

PACING UP

It is really important that you start with a manageable amount of activity – an amount that you are comfortable and confident with – and slowly increase this as your fitness improves. This is called pacing up.

Remember Jim with the arthritis in his knees? When he came to my clinic in a state of despair, I talked to him about his doctor's advice. It was, indeed, good for him to do short walks to increase the strength and stability of his knees. Once he understood that what he'd been doing was harmful, we developed a helpful graduated program. He started off with short walks, even though walking wasn't the most comfortable thing for him. Jim persevered because he now better understood the need to stay active. To build on his start, Jim gradually increased the distance and speed of his walks. Even when he wasn't feeling the best and his knees ached, he stuck to his plan by pacing himself and gradually building up his fitness. Jim also routinely used an ice pack after his walk, both to give himself some relief and to help distract his brain from the pain messages. Every day, it became a bit better. Even when he felt like going further than he should, Jim reminded himself that slow and steady wins the race. When the lawn looked untidy again, Jim pushed his old lawn mower around his big backyard, but instead of doing it all in one go, he finished half then left the other half for the next day. Over time he slowly increased what he could do. Jim felt more positive and confident about his rehabilitation, and he could *feel* the difference in this new moderate well-paced approach. There was definitely light at the end of the tunnel.

Getting off the Rollercoaster

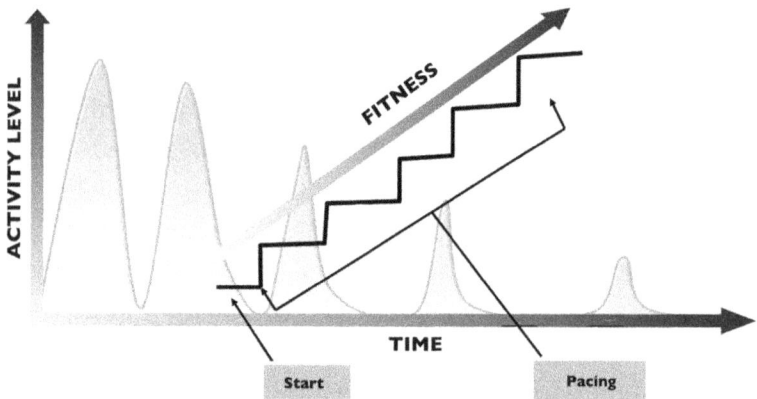

Pacing up: this diagram shows that over time, fitness increases when activity increases.

Even if you have been on the overactivity–underactivity rollercoaster, your future pain management can change if you adopt the more helpful method of pacing up. When people hear of this method to manage their pain, a common reaction is self-blame: *I should have known better. I should have realised.* But those thoughts are not helpful and they don't change anything. The important thing is that you see a new way, and give it a go.

When I first started my training for the trek to the Mt Everest base camp, I really pushed myself. Once, I got a little over-enthusiastic, donned my hiking gear, loaded my back-pack to 10 kg, and went to climb the 1,000 steps at the base of Mt Dandenong. It was 4.30 am one winter's day. It was dark and cold, but that didn't stop me. With my torch in one hand and a walking stick in the other, I went up and down three times. It was okay while I was doing it, but because I didn't pace myself, I experienced a delayed pain response.

Not only did I suffer for about a week afterwards, but the resulting pain almost made me consider quitting my quest to trek to the Mt Everest base camp. I really beat myself up about it too, especially since I *should* have known better.

While I was experiencing the pain in the days after my over-activity, I realised just how easy it is to become complacent, even when you know the right way to do things. Even though I should have known better, I challenged my unhelpful thoughts and considered the bigger picture: I had loaded my back-pack, I had made the effort to drive out to Mt Dandenong, and I had climbed the steps in an effort to train for my trek. All these were good helpful things. The only thing I had done wrong was to be a little too enthusiastic, which, of course, is human nature. What I was doing was right; I just needed to pace myself.

I use my own experience to remind my clients that, while reaching your destination is important, so is the journey that takes you there. Don't be too hard on yourself. Pace yourself, and enjoy your journey. You'll learn a lot about yourself along the way.

ADVANTAGES AND DISADVANTAGES OF PACING UP

So why aren't pacing techniques used more often? People are often scared of the pain. They believe that pain necessitates rest. Take a look at the following advantages and disadvantages. This just might change your mind.

Advantages	Disadvantages
• You have a manageable starting point from which you can build on.	• Your progress might be slow at first.
• You will be able to achieve your goals.	• You may become impatient with the pace of your gradual build-up of activity and fitness.
• You can also incorporate things you enjoy into your plan.	• You may get frustrated if you can't complete things in one go.
• You feel a sense of achievement and control as you make gains.	• You may feel disappointed at the starting point because it seems low compared to what you used to be able to do.
• You will be able to see your progress clearly.	• You may be worried or anxious about doing something new, or not have faith it will work.
• You will become more independent and be able to plan things in advance.	• You may be nervous about the increased expectations others will have of you once they see you improve.

- You will feel more useful and other people will see you as a capable person.

- Your confidence will grow and your mood will improve.

- You will be able to do more things socially and have more to talk about than just your pain.

- You are in control of your pain, and not the other way around.

- You will be fitter and healthier, despite your pain.

Thankfully, the disadvantages of pacing are short-term, but in the longer-term, there is a bigger, more promising picture. Pacing allows you to achieve your goals without the struggle. It allows you to recover faster and feel more rejuvenated. Pacing allows you to enjoy the experience and build confidence in your ability to manage your pain. It is the best option. But remember, some of this is about trial and error, and if you don't get it right the first time, don't beat yourself up about it.

Of course, making changes can be challenging, but it helps to focus on the bigger picture and work towards it. If looking at the bigger picture feels overwhelming and a long way off, remember the old saying: *a journey of a thousand miles begins with a single step.*

Use the difficult times you have had in the past and learn from them. Turn the negative experiences to learning experiences. Learn from your mistakes, just like I have.

WHEN THINGS ARE GOING WELL

When things start to go well for you, don't suddenly change your plans. Don't try and do more, no matter how tempting it is. Stick to your plans, and gradually increase the pace, week by week. Continue to take breaks, use heat/ice packs if they help, or whatever is part of your pacing strategy. If you feel good and continue to pace yourself, your body will be grateful because you are allowing it to operate at an optimal level, not a maximum level. You are also allowing your body to recover faster. Not only that, you will be able to keep going with fewer flare-ups of pain. It's all about pacing and sticking to a plan.

Whenever I talk about pacing with my clients, I often remember the time when my mate Chan took me out for a movie and a few drinks. I felt great being at the movies, and even better because I was out and about. Of course, the right thing to do was to call it a night – a good night – straight after the movie. Temptation got the better of me, and I stayed out. And my body paid for it. It was a great reminder of the importance of staying focused and pacing yourself.

PRESSURE

By nature, people are competitive. You may be tempted to compare yourself with others in similar circumstances and look at what they have achieved. It is important to remember that everyone is different, and that everyone should have different goals and time-frames. Some people don't compete with others, but instead compete with what they used to be able to do. Remember that you are trying to work out what is manageable for you at the present time, not what you managed in the past or what you think you should be able to manage. Unnecessary pressure or stress will only keep the lights green on the pain highway.

Recognise that any step now, no matter how small, is a significant improvement on before.

THOUGHTS AND EMOTIONS

People may not realise how their thoughts and feelings affect their pain levels. The mind and the body work together; everything is connected. People who have a helpful, positive mindset actually feel less pain. This chapter looks at helpful and unhelpful thinking patterns, and explains the importance of understanding the mind-body-pain connection.

HOW OUR THINKING AFFECTS US

One of the biggest factors in the management of chronic pain is the way the person thinks about it.

Imagine that two people are suffering from the same level of chronic pain. One person gets angry, frustrated and anxious, and is quick to blame the pain: *I can't even walk down the road because of my pain.* The second person has a different way of thinking about their pain: *this pain is frustrating, but at least I'm able to walk down the street.* This person feels more positive about their progress and know that, if they manage their pain properly, they will be fine.

Which person do you think experiences less pain?

Of course, it is the second person who is managing their pain with a more positive approach.

Both have the same pain, but the one major difference is how they *think* about their pain.

Let's look at this in another way. You're at a scary movie and there's a scene where a young woman turns the door knob to go inside her apartment, unaware of the serial killer standing behind the louvers in her bedroom cupboard. Your heart starts to pound, your hair stands on end and your body tenses up. You are scared of what is about to happen. But why are you scared?

Is it the movie?

Or is it your *thoughts* about what is about to happen that scare you?

Of course, it is your thoughts. You know how these things go. The music is dramatic and creepy, the shadows showing the killer's eyes through the louvers sends chills up your spine, the dramatic build-up and the young woman's innocence. Not to mention your background understanding gained from every horror movie you've ever watched. The physical movie – the screen, the moving images and the music – can't hurt you. It is your *thoughts* that cause the spine-tingling and heart-racing responses.

The fact that our thoughts can drive how we feel physically and emotionally may be a new understanding for you. To help make more sense of this, let's look at a couple of more examples.

Imagine you just sat an important test. You walk away *thinking* that you failed. How would you feel? You're probably stressed, upset, frustrated and disappointed. You may sweat, feel fatigued and even feel a little sick.

Now imagine you sat the same important test, and answered the questions exactly the same as before. But this time you walked away *thinking* you passed. How would you feel? You're probably happy, joyful and ecstatic. Your body may be full of adrenaline; you feel awake and ready to celebrate.

Can you see that, despite writing the same answers on the test, the way you *think* about it afterwards can have a significant effect on how you feel both emotionally and physically?

Our thoughts absolutely affect how we feel.

Let's take another example, this time with knee pain.
Sarah is a 35-year-old accountant who enjoys walking and
jogging. For a few years now, she has had knee pain and
is getting increasingly frustrated and anxious about her
persisting pain. One day, she goes for a walk and her knee
pain increases. This increase makes her angry, frustrated
and upset. She can't believe that her knee still plays up.
She blames her walking and decides to go back home. Her
heart starts to race and she starts to feel tense; the pain is
really affecting her.

Now consider a slightly different scenario. Sarah has
had knee pain for a while and this pain increases one day
when she goes for a walk. Despite the discomfort and some
frustration, she remains positive as she can see the progress
she has made. She thinks in a more helpful manner, paces
herself and continues with her walk. Her heart rate is a
little high but her tension levels are managed and the pain
is not so bad.

There is something interesting to note here. The same
situation, knee pain while walking, has elicited very
different feelings and behaviours. What do you think Sarah
is thinking for her to be so upset, angry and frustrated?
Perhaps:

- *I can't get rid of this pain.*
- *I hate my pain.*
- *I'll never go walking again.*

What do you think Sarah is thinking for her to have
some frustration, but generally remain in a more positive
frame of mind? Perhaps:

- *At least I am walking more now and I can get out of
  the house.*

- *The pain is frustrating but if I continue to pace myself, I'll be able to do this.*
- *This is something I will learn to manage, so I can move on.*

Which thoughts do you think are more helpful for Sarah? Which thoughts do you think would help her manage her symptoms? Putting it into a diagram, it would look like this:

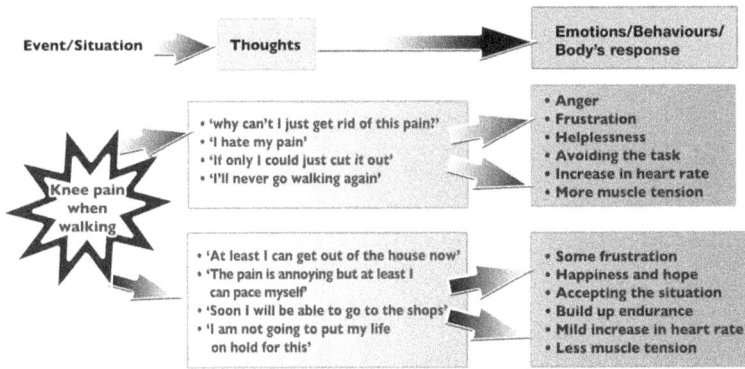

Event/Situation → Thoughts → Emotions/Behaviours/ Body's response

Knee pain when walking

- 'why can't I just get rid of this pain?'
- 'I hate my pain'
- 'If only I could just cut it out'
- 'I'll never go walking again'

- Anger
- Frustration
- Helplessness
- Avoiding the task
- Increase in heart rate
- More muscle tension

- 'At least I can get out of the house now'
- 'The pain is annoying but at least I can pace myself'
- 'Soon I will be able to go to the shops'
- 'I am not going to put my life on hold for this'

- Some frustration
- Happiness and hope
- Accepting the situation
- Build up endurance
- Mild increase in heart rate
- Less muscle tension

How your thoughts affect your emotions and behaviours

This example shows that, for any given situation, your thoughts can have a significant effect on how you feel, how you behave and how your body responds. It's not just the situation you find yourself in. If you have unhelpful thoughts, you tend to end up in an unhelpful, and often negative, frame of mind. An unhelpful frame of mind leads to unhelpful behaviour, and the pain traffic lights stay green. The opposite occurs when you have helpful or positive thoughts. You accept your pain, you believe in your abilities to take control of your pain and the pain traffic lights turn red; you move on.

Don't fall into the trap of thinking that pushing through

your pain is being positive. This may be a positive attitude, but being positive in this way isn't helpful in the longer term. Remember the overactivity–underactivity rollercoaster. Effective pain management is not about pushing through the pain at all. A more helpful way of thinking is: *I'll pace myself and build-up gradually*. This is still being positive, but in a more helpful way.

AUTOMATIC THINKING

Thoughts run through your mind all the time, most of which you are not conscious of. You walk downstairs each morning and never pay attention to the action of descending one step at a time, one foot after another, how fast you are going to go, or how confident you are doing it. All this happens without any conscious thought from you. These thoughts are called automatic thoughts and we don't even realise that we have them. Automatic thoughts are normal, but if your automatic thoughts become mostly unhelpful and negative – often without you realising – they can actually accentuate your pain levels and start to work against you.

MAKING THE LINKS

Every clinician regularly hears patients say that their pain increases in intensity when they're in an unhelpful frame of mind – when they are arguing with family, worrying about their future, or feeling anxious about their pain. You might be familiar with some of the most common thoughts:

- *What have I done to deserve this?*
- *Why me?*
- *I will never be happy.*
- *This pain is killing me.*

These thoughts lead to feelings of sadness, helplessness,

worry and anger. If people understood the extent to which these thoughts cause physical changes in their bodies – faster heartbeat, sweaty palms, clamminess and tense muscles – and realised that these thoughts caused their pain traffic lights to remain green, they would put as much effort into their mind as they put into their body.

As much as your thoughts affect how you feel and behave, your emotions and behaviour, in turn, affects your thoughts. They all feed off one another and are independent of the situation.

Going back to the above example, even if Sarah's knee pain subsided, if she had adopted a negative mindset, she would still be upset, she would still avoid activity and this would lead to more unhelpful thoughts. Put into a diagram, it would look like this:

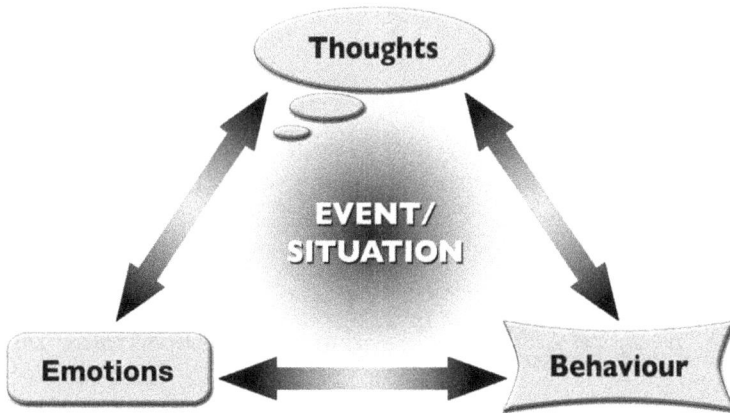

How our thoughts, behaviour, and emotions interact

The more unhelpful your state of mind, the more pain you feel.

Let's explore the most common emotions of people with chronic pain. If we understand them, we can recognise and address them.

ANGER

Anger is an emotion that everyone feels. It is a normal emotion and, at times, can be useful. Anger at an injustice can pump us full of adrenaline and call us to action. If we saw a bunch of teenagers taunting a scared old lady, we would use our anger and do something about it. It can make us feel fired up and rearing to go.

When people with chronic pain feel anger at their situation, it is really counter-productive. In extreme cases, anger can lead to aggression and violence. Not only that, but it also releases chemicals that keep the pain traffic lights on green, and anger can actually make an angry person feel more pain.

Angry thoughts	Helpful thoughts
I shouldn't have vacuumed the whole house in one go!	*I could do half today and half tomorrow.*
They should understand how I'm feeling!	*I could help them understand how I'm feeling. At least they are trying to help.*
I should be able to kick a footy with the kids!	*It is frustrating that I can't do this now, but I am doing something about it.*

ANXIETY

We all become anxious at times. Back when we were cavemen, anxiety helped keep us safe and prevented us from taking unnecessary risks. Picture a caveman sitting in his cave. He hears a noise which makes him anxious and alert. Is it a threat? His anxiety means that he can't ignore it, and it keeps him prepared. At low levels, anxiety looks like simple cautiousness – don't spill the hot cup of tea, be careful going down the stairs. At high levels, anxiety takes over and stops us from problem solving and dealing with the tasks in front of us.

Picture a student so anxious that he forgets exam questions, or a mother so anxious that her child will get hurt that she is incapable of enjoying being a mother. People with chronic pain commonly worry about their pain levels increasing or maybe that they are doing further damage. They worry that they won't be able to handle things any more. They worry about not being able to provide for their family. They worry that other people won't understand their pain. This constant worry doesn't help. In fact, it causes more pain.

Anxious thoughts	Helpful thoughts
What if my pain gets worse?	*If my pain does get worse, I will pace myself better.*
What if I cause more damage?	*I have a better understanding of my pain and I know that I am not doing more damage.*
Will I ever get better?	*People with pain can live a normal life.*

LOW MOOD AND DEPRESSION

When someone suffers from chronic pain, a lot more can be lost than just their pain-free past. They may lose their job, independence, relationships, financial security, good health, and the inability to achieve their goals and desires. In fact, it can feel like they have lost everything. This loss can lead to sufferers feeling low and depressed.

In life, things happen that make us feel sad or low, but

for most of us, these feelings usually go away after a while and our mood never moves from low to depressed. However, if these feelings go on for a long time, you may start to imagine that things will never improve and your future starts looking very bleak. If a person gets stuck in this bleak reality, they can become depressed. And, not surprisingly, someone who has lost the most important things in their life will feel wretched.

If the pain is not dealt with, a downward spiral is almost inevitable. Feeling low will keep the pain traffic lights on green and increase the pain.

Low thoughts	Helpful thoughts
I'll never be able to dance again.	*I might not be able to do that now, but I can work up to it.*
I can't even jog for 10 minutes.	*I can jog for five minutes now. I will continue to pace and aim to jog for 10 minutes in about four weeks.*
If only I didn't have this pain, I could live a normal life.	*People with pain can live a normal life.*

DISTORTED THINKING PATTERNS

If a person is in an unhelpful mindset most of the time, they will see things in a distorted way. This might involve:

- All-or-nothing thinking – Things appear only as black-or-white or right-or-wrong, with no grey areas. Example: *I will either vacuum the whole house, or not do it at all.*
- Over-generalisation – You generalise a single

negative event as a never-ending pattern of defeat or failure. Examples: *I'm always going to struggle to wash the car* and *I'll never be the same again.*

- Mental filter – You use one incident or aspect of a situation to view the entire situation in a negative way. Example: *My daily walks take longer than usual because of my pain, and it takes away the whole enjoyment of doing it.*

- Discounting the positive – You reject positive experiences or achievements, insisting that they don't count. Example: *Being able to wash the car doesn't really count because I can't do it as often as I used to be able to.*

- Mind reading – You assume that you know what other people are thinking, without actually knowing for sure. Example: *People think I am faking it because they can't see my pain.*

- Fortune telling – You make predictions about the way things will work out. Example: *If I try and pick that off the floor, my discs will pop out.*

- Personalisation – You assume that things are your fault and you take responsibility for things that are out of your control. Example: *It was my fault that the house wasn't clean when your mother dropped in the other day. I should have cleaned up.*

- Catastrophizing – You see negative events that will occur in the future as catastrophic and come up with worst case scenarios. Example: *I will end up in a wheelchair if I'm not careful.*

- Labelling – You attach a negative label to yourself as a result of a situation. Example: *I'm a failure because I can't support my family.*

Do you hear yourself in any of the examples above? Have a think about your self-talk. Become more aware of your internal dialogue. You may be guilty of labelling yourself in a negative way. You may be guilty of imagining worst case scenarios. And most of us are guilty of all-or-nothing thinking.

The problem is that it doesn't matter what practical things you do in response to an increase in pain, if your thoughts aren't helpful, you are going to suffer more pain. So, if you recognise yourself in any of the above examples, make an effort to change your thinking. Challenge unhelpful thoughts and replace them with more helpful ones. Then you can begin to use your thoughts to work for you, not against you.

Some people find that, in the heat of the moment when they are most angry or upset, they can't even think straight, let alone challenge any unhelpful thinking. The area of the brain that deals with our emotion dates back to primitive days. When our emotions are heightened, we can tend to act not much differently to the days when we lived in caves and had to run from woolly mammoths. Fight or flight. In times of great anger or frustration, the logic centre in our brains can actually be taken over by the more primal response centre.

Just as our mind can play tricks on us, we too can play tricks on our mind. If you feel yourself getting into unhelpful thinking that you can't seem to get out of, you can simply find a quiet place to calm down.

Breathe deeply.

Relax.

Picture a place that makes you feel calm.

See the beauty of this place.

Breathe deeply.

What thoughts were going through your mind at the time?

What would be a more helpful way of thinking?

Makes you feel better just reading it, doesn't it? Your thought centre and your emotion centre are in constant communication with each other. It is your thoughts that regulate your emotions. When we are really angry, frustrated, or depressed, the emotional area takes over, and that's why we often find we just can't think straight, no matter how hard we try. During these times, you need to take deep breaths and practice relaxation skills to get your emotions under control. Research shows that calm deep breathing helps to take the edge off intense emotions, allowing you to take back some control and think helpfully again. This is why we can think and reflect once we have had time to calm down.

THE HEALING PROCESS

Many doctors treat chronic pain as if it is acute pain. If you understand the healing process, you will see why this approach does not work. At each stage of the healing process, different things happen in your body and require different treatments. This chapter explores each stage of the healing process, what is happening to you, and how you can respond.

STAGES OF HEALING

Many people only have a rudimentary knowledge about how to treat themselves in the event of injury. It can be confusing knowing when to use ice-packs, bandages, straps, heat-packs, bandaids, gauze, Betadine and aspirin. The reality is that, if you manage your injury well in its early stages, there is less likelihood of the pain turning chronic.

To know how to treat injuries, we need to have an understanding of the body's healing process. There are four stages of healing:
- the inflammatory stage
- the repair stage
- the contraction stage
- the remodelling stage.

Understanding these stages will help you know what needs to be done during each stage to minimise pain and maximise healing.

INFLAMMATORY STAGE

When we first injure ourselves, tissue is damaged. Damaged tissue discharges chemicals that cause the release of Serous fluid. Serous fluid is the clear, sticky stuff that comes out of a blister. The thickness and stickiness of the serous fluid is due to a protein called collagen. The collagen forms a plug, or a clot, to stop the bleeding.

Although inflammation is an important part of the healing process, too much inflammation results in healthy tissue also being stuck together by the serous fluid, and this isn't good for the healthy tissues. Just say you banged your shin on the coffee table. Without intervention, the injured part will swell up much more than is actually needed for healing. Instead of the serous fluid just clotting the immediate tissue area and blocking the damaged blood vessels, the serous fluid builds up and moves to the surrounding muscles, ligaments and nerves. The problem is that the serous fluid is like superglue; you only need a little to stick things together, a whole blob will end up also sticking other things that you don't want stuck together.

THE RICE PRINCIPLE

In treating an acute injury properly, we often use the RICE principle.

> R = Relative Rest or Relative Movement
> I = Ice
> C = Compression
> E = Elevation

R = Relative rest or Relative movement

There has been a lot of misunderstanding about what the letter R stands for. Too often it is referred to as just *Rest*, but this is not what good medical practitioners recommend because rest is often counter-productive to healing. Introducing some gentle movement early on helps in many ways. Firstly, it promotes circulation to remove any excess serous fluid and bruising. Secondly, it maintains the health of undamaged tissues by keeping them mobile. If you keep still, the swelling increases and the body part often becomes stiff and more painful. Gentle movement also has a dulling effect on the pain because it gives the brain something else to focus on besides the pain. A good example of this is when you jam your finger in a door. You instinctively shake the fingers vigorously which divides your brain's focus.

Interesting....
Some of the fastest bones to heal following a fracture are your ribs. Ribs heal extremely fast because they are constantly moving in a gentle manner, encouraging the healing process to take place quickly.

With most injuries, particularly with sprains and strains, and even most fractures, the importance of movement, especially gentle movement, is vital early in the recovery process. In most cases, relative rest, not complete rest, is what is important. Immobilising an injury completely should be restricted to conditions like an unstable fracture, skin graft or a venomous bite.

Take a moment to also consider what time of day you would find the most painful following an injury. Most people say that it is when they first wake up. When you sleep, the body is not as physically active and there is less circulation, which means that swelling sets in, nerves become sensitive, and there is less information to distract the brain and dull the pain. However, following a warm shower and gentle movements, the pain tends to ease. People often say that during the day, the pain appears to be better than at night or early in the mornings. This is because, during the day, you generally move more, improve circulation and also distract the brain.

The notion of doctors ordering complete bed rest for anything is obsolete – well, apart from a very few conditions. Prolonged bed rest has a two-fold effect. Firstly, the inflammation results in healthy tissues being stuck together, and secondly, a lack of movement means that the brain maintains the pain traffic lights on green and the patient feels more pain.

I = Ice

When we injure ourselves, we use ice to slow down the swelling and manage the pain by numbing the area. The brain is partially distracted from the pain because it has to process cold information as well as pain.

It is important to wait about five minutes after an injury before introducing a cold-pack. This allows time for some serous fluid to be released into the area, but ensures that not too much is released. It also slows the blood flowing from the damaged blood vessels, decreasing the size of the resulting bruise.

C = Compression

Compression is helpful with ice because it provides external pressure to contain the serous fluid to the injured area. Effective compression is only possible using an appropriate pressure bandage. Don't use Tubi-grip or crepe bandages because these have high elasticity and can't be applied firmly enough. When applying compression, you need to ensure that any grooves around the affected body part, such as the grooves around the ankle, are filled with cotton before the pressure bandage is put on. This is necessary to ensure that there is even pressure and that there are no gaps for the swelling to move to when compression is applied.

E = Elevation

By elevating the injured body part above the level of the heart, gravity can be used to assist the circulation to bring the swelling back towards the heart, and then remove it. The problem is that often people don't realise that the elevated body part, whether it is a wrist or an ankle, needs to be above the level of the heart for this to work effectively. Too often people just sit up with their ankle on a foot rest or pillow; they need to lie down so that they can raise the ankle above the level of the heart.

This inflammatory stage occurs within ten minutes of the injury and in most cases, lasts from two to ten days. For this reason, anti-inflammatory tablets will only be effective within that time period. The persistent swelling that occurs with most chronic pain conditions, such as chronic regional pain syndrome (or repetitive strain injury) and fibromyalgia, isn't due to ongoing injury or damage, but due to changes in the tissues and circulation.

REPAIR STAGE

The repair stage starts within two to three days of the injury. During this time, the clot forms a scar. When the scar tissue is formed, it is formed in a disorganised way, like a weak clump.

Studies have shown that scar tissue doesn't really respond to anything but movement. With movement, the clumps of scar tissue fibres begin to align, repair and strengthen. With an ankle injury, for example, you need to identify all the directions that your ankle can move and then incorporate these movements into a gentle exercise routine. This allows the scar to be stretched so the tissue can align appropriately. Complete rest of an injured ankle would result in it becoming stiff, swollen, painful and weak.

The repair stage typically finishes within one week for minor injuries like a cut finger, and within three months for any serious injury. If there are no complications, all injuries will be healed within three months, no matter how severe. Any pain that persists after three months is not a sign of further damage or injury, but is the result of changes in the sensitivity of your nerves.

CONTRACTION STAGE

Within two weeks following an injury, scars begins to tighten and contract to bind the edges of a wound together. Gentle stretching is needed early on to prevent over-tightness. Burns victims are taught stretches and self-massage early to encourage elasticity in their skin.

Even with a typical back strain, after the inflammatory and repair phases, the scar will begin to shrink and put tension on the tissues. If you have been immobile, when you try to move, you are likely to feel an immediate jabbing pain as the tissues pull on one another.

Therefore, to maximise the benefits of the contraction stage, gentle stretching and movement is needed.

REMODELLING STAGE

Remodelling is when the scar tissue forms into a state close to that of the original tissue. It is never too late for this remodelling to occur. Remodelling can occur for years, and can start at any time. People who have had terrible scars can begin stretches, massage and exercises years later to help remodel the tissues. These people have reported great successes.

Because your body is constantly rejuvenating – replacing old tissue with new tissue – it is never too late to start. Even if you have been told that you have scar tissue, think about that body part and what it normally does and gently increase its range of movement to help the remodelling process.

KEEPING OUR BODIES HEALTHY AND STRONG

From the time when *Homo sapiens* first roamed the land, their bodies have adapted. Being active has always been the key to a healthy lifestyle. In the past, activity was part of life. Today, this is not the case for a lot of people. This chapter explores how your body can adapt to your lifestyle choices, and what is needed to keep your body healthy and strong.

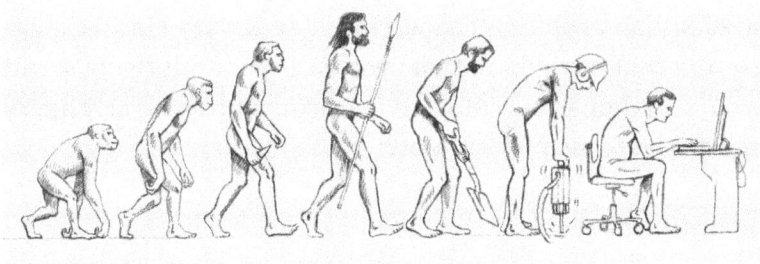

Human evolution

ADAPTING

From the tree-climbing creatures of the early days to what we are today, evolutionary change has been affected by environmental factors and our lifestyle choices. Our bodies are amazing. If you train yourself to stand in one spot for hours like the guards at Buckingham Palace, you can do it. You can train yourself to somersault from a highwire, run a marathon, climb mountains or swim the English Channel.

In fact, given enough time, your body will adapt to almost anything you put it through. To have an understanding of where we are headed, let's take a brief look at evolution.

Hunter-gatherers

Around three or four million years ago, we were hunters and gatherers; the fittest survived and the weak didn't. People were always on the move, had plenty of exercise and food was plentiful. Men climbed trees, hunted for food and carried their bounty tens of kilometres back to their camp site. The women gathered food and protected the young. To survive, they needed to be strong, fit and agile.

Interestingly, research suggests that about 150,000 years ago, our species was close to extinction. It is estimated that, at one point, the number of people in the whole world may have dwindled down to as low as 10,000. This is based on research that shows that the genetic make-up of the seven or so billion people in the world today is very similar, suggesting that our population evolved from a relatively small group. Perhaps this could be a reason why some strangers remind us of people we know.

Agricultural revolution

Approximately 13,000 years ago, the agricultural revolution began. People settled into permanent communities. There was no longer a need to regularly migrate, nor was there such a great need for hunting. They started to grow and harvest foods depending on the seasons. Their duties and tasks also varied depending on the seasons. The men tended to animals and crops, and there was less variety in their tasks. The working week was up to 70 hours long. Generally, the people of this era were strong and fit, but slightly less agile because they were doing the same tasks over and over.

Industrial revolution

In the late 1700s, the industrial revolution not only changed the way society worked, but it changed people's physical activity levels. As people began to depend on machines, physical exertion lessened. Life was lived in one place, the variety of physical tasks decreased, and people became less strong, fit and agile.

Modern times

In a complete turnabout from our ancestors, we now have machines to perform most of the tasks that used to be done by hand or hard labour. Now, many people need to join gyms to get the physical activity required for good health.

REVERSING HISTORY

So what do we need to do to keep our bodies healthy and strong?

Exercises and stretches

Ligaments, muscles and tendons are kept healthy with regular stretching and exercise. Having good flexibility and fitness makes injury less likely, and the endorphins released by exercise make you feel good and help turn pain traffic lights to red. Exercise is good for your heart and circulation, your lung capacity and bone strength, and it keeps your skin healthy and elastic: all good things.

Remember these simple facts:
- your heart is a muscle that needs exercise just like any other muscle
- exercise improves your lungs by increasing their capacity – the deeper you breathe, the more oxygen circulates through your body

- increased oxygen and blood flow carry more nutrients to your skin – hence the healthy glow people often have after exercising
- exercise improves muscle tone and strength – if you have a weak knee and you build up your leg muscles, then they can help support the knee
- bones are kept healthy by having pressure put through them – when we move, blood is pushed out of the bone and when we take the pressure off, blood is sucked back in. This in and out movement of blood keeps our bones healthy
- exercise keeps joints healthy – movement releases a thin film of lubricating fluid inside the joint that contains nutrients which are good for the cartilage
- better circulation increases blood flow to the brain, improving concentration and memory
- mood, sleep and your immune system all benefit from exercise
- exercise and movement help your digestive system
- exercise helps to reduce traffic on the pain highway

Just before the petrol bomb attack, I was fit and healthy and ready to complete a 10 km fun-run. When I was stuck at home during my rehabilitation, I lost my energy, my enthusiasm, and couldn't even remember what it felt like to be happy and positive.

It was a real eye opener for me.

The best thing I did was to sort out a rehabilitation program. When I started, it was difficult. I was in pain and I felt stiff. The road ahead seemed long.

But I needed to start somewhere.

Before long, the stretches and exercises helped improve the condition of my skin and my body. I felt fitter, and this allowed me to get back to the things I enjoyed doing.

I could once again focus on my goal of getting to the Mount Everest base camp. The exercises improved my sleep. No more nights were spent staring at the ceiling, wondering if I would ever recover. A better night's sleep meant I was refreshed and rejuvenated.

Relaxation techniques

Over the years, relaxation techniques have become widely used. Actors and elite athletes use relaxation techniques to calm themselves before a performance or event. Military marksmen use relaxation techniques to concentrate on their heart rates, allowing them to pull the trigger in between heartbeats. We often use these techniques without even realising it. Think about the calming breaths you might take before you give a big presentation at work. Or when standing in front of goal posts, ready to kick the goal that will decide the outcome of a game; you steady yourself, take a deep breath and release it slowly before you kick.

Relaxation techniques, like those discussed later in the Beyond Pain program, help us to relax our minds and allow tension and anxiety to flow from our bodies.

Tension causes pain so it is important to develop techniques that release tension. For some people – particularly men – the thought of using a relaxation technique may not be appealing, but it *is* a powerful strategy that can give you relief from pain and tension.

When you have a flare-up of pain, stretching and exercising might be the last things you feel like doing. Relaxation techniques can help get your pain levels under control, help turn the pain traffic lights to red and get you back on track. Remember, it is not about pushing through your pain, it is about learning to manage it effectively. Relaxation techniques can also replace medications, or at least help reduce medication levels.

A good night's sleep

Having a good night's sleep will refresh you, replenish your energy levels, reduce your pain, improve your mood and keep your appetite healthy. Yet, so many people with chronic pain report difficulty with sleeping.

There are many research studies that show how sleep affects pain levels. One study of nearly one thousand adult chronic pain sufferers showed that a poor night's sleep resulted in increased pain levels the following day.

Relaxation techniques such as those discussed in the Beyond Pain program can be used to reduce the tension in your body and calm your mind before going to bed, to ensure a better night's sleep.

SCANS AND X-RAYS: WHAT THEY CAN AND CAN'T SHOW

Scans and x-rays come with their own terminology. Words like 'degenerative' and 'broad-based disc-bulge' are used and often scare people who don't understand what these terms really mean. This chapter explores what scans and x-rays actually show us and examines the terminology that doctors use.

SEEKING THE ANSWER

When we feel pain, it is in our nature to find out why. We want a diagnosis for it and then try to get rid of it. Commonly, there is peace of mind when we get our diagnosis, even if it is vague. When the diagnosis comes, people say, 'Well, at least I know what it is.'

Scans and x-rays are often used to get these diagnoses. When we are dealing with acute pain, having scans and x-rays can be very beneficial. Following a thorough assessment, these investigations can be used to confirm a diagnosis beyond any doubt and give the patient the peace of mind they are looking for.

Scans and x-rays can also assist in the treatment of some chronic pain conditions. They are used as aids during surgery to help remove cancers and they help guide doctors when they inject pain medications into a joint or a muscle.

Scans and x-rays certainly can play a vital role in the treatment of acute pain.

But some people don't understand that scans themselves are not treatments. Some people come into my clinic feeling disappointed that they're not feeling better after a full round of tests. Conversations go something like this:

Patient: I had the MRI scan last week, but I'm still in a lot of pain.

Me: What were you expecting?

Patient: I thought it might help, show something at least ... I don't know.

Most people, particularly those with chronic pain, visit many specialists for x-rays, ultrasounds, CT scans, MRIs and nerve conduction tests. Sometimes doctors suggest a repeat of these tests after a flare-up of pain. But the reality is that, if a diagnosis has been made, more scans won't change anything. The focus should be on the management and treatment of the pain.

Think about it; if you have a bulging disc and get a scan of your back during a flare-up and compare it to a scan taken on a better day, you will see your bulging disc in both scans. So what is making the pain better and worse? It can't be the disc. Remember the pain traffic lights in the spinal cord? The flare-up could be due to stress or anger, but scans can't show this. And anyway, will another scan change the way you manage your pain?

Unfortunately, people with chronic pain sometimes willingly endure more pain and suffering having these tests, just to get a diagnosis. Some spend thousands and thousands of dollars on tests that often don't come up with a diagnosis. These tests may stretch over many years, and they may delay treatments that will help in the long-term.

Around two-thirds of my clients have no discernible

reason for their pain, which means that all the tests they've had don't show clearly what is wrong or why. Generally speaking, when it comes to chronic pain, there is limited benefit in having repeated scans and x-rays.

I always ask clients, 'What matters most – finding a diagnosis for your chronic pain, or improving your situation and moving on?'

NOT CALLING A SPADE A SPADE

As we get older, our skin wrinkles, our hair becomes grey and our bones age too. Bones lose calcium, and arthritis starts to set-in. This is normal. Most people, from their early twenties onwards, will show some age-related changes, particularly in their discs, bones and joints. Unfortunately, most x-ray reports describe these changes as *degenerative*, implying that there is something wrong. Health practitioners call these changes degenerative because, in most cases, this is the way age-related changes are described in medical terms. Of course, there are circumstances such as following trauma and in some congenital cases, when degeneration occurs early in life. But in general, the term 'degenerative' is used to describe normal age-related change. Unfortunately, patients hear the word 'degenerative' and panic.

One of my patients was told he had degenerative disc disease. He had tried the typical physiotherapy and chiropractic treatments and nothing had helped. When he came to me, distressed by his diagnosis, I explained that, in his case, it was just another way of saying that his discs were ageing normally. His pain wasn't because of his *degenerative discs* but because of over-sensitive nerves in his body.

Once my patient learned that his discs were normal for his age, and understood about his over-sensitive nerves and the strategies that would help, his thinking about his pain changed. Previously he had been fearful of activity, but he now embraced the stretches and exercises, and went back to the things he enjoyed doing. It took him a bit of time to adjust, but he re-wrote his truths. The change was amazing. The man who had first shuffled into my clinic looking about 30 years older than he was, now moved more confidently, had a spring in his step and looked a lot younger. He was living a much better life in just four weeks. Ironically, his next scan was much the same as his original one.

When your discs are ageing normally, some therapists refer to it as a degenerative disease, but it's like calling grey hair a degenerative hair disease. Or like calling wrinkles a degenerative skin disease. In medical terms, it probably makes sense, but the phrase 'degenerative disease' always frightens people.

Therapists have lots of complicated terms for things that are completely normal, or for things that they don't actually understand. One phrase that strikes fear into the hearts of pain sufferers is *chronic musculoskeletal pain syndrome* (translation: chronic pain in the muscles and bones). Another common term is *fibromyalgia*, which literally translates into 'aches in the muscles and tissues'. So, in fact, the patient goes to the doctor saying that they have aches in their muscles and tissues, and their doctor does some tests and comes back with a diagnosis that they have aches in their muscles and tissues.

Another issue that arises from scans and x-rays is that often a disc bulge is shown and is immediately diagnosed as the cause of the pain. It is also immediately assumed that disc bulges squash the nerves. But in most cases, this doesn't happen. In fact, most people over the age of 25 years have at least one bulging disc and experience no pain at all.

Fortunately, in recent times, health practitioners are beginning to use more helpful descriptions such as *disc bulge consistent with age-related changes*, which are far less scary, and describe the changes more accurately.

Consider the following excerpt from a report:

CT SCAN - LUMBOSACRAL SPINE:

Axial scans with thin slices were performed. Reformatted images were then provided.

Only mild broad based posterior disc bulge is seen at L5/S1. The thecal sac and nerve roots are preserved at all levels.

No evidence of focal disc herniation, central spinal canal stenosis, or nerve root impingement is detected.

No pars defect or slipping is seen.

Conclusion: No signficant abnormality is seen.

The radiologist describes a broad-based disc bulge and reports no significant abnormality – because in this case it is completely normal

WHAT SCANS CAN'T SHOW

Advances in scans and x-rays have led us to the diagnosis and treatment of more medical conditions than ever before. We are now able to see inside our bodies with an unprecedented level of detail and accuracy. Today, we can see babies smile inside the womb using 4-dimensional ultrasounds, and watch the brain working using functional MRIs.

Although scans and x-rays can show a lot, they can't always show the exact cause of the pain. They can't show when you are in pain, and they can't show actual pain.

Just imagine you lift something heavy and experience a sudden sharp pain in your back. Your doctor sends you for a scan which shows a bulging disc and a muscle strain. How do you know what is causing you pain just by looking at the scan? Is it the disc? Or is it the strain? Could it be both? How do you know that the bulging disc and the muscle strain weren't there earlier? You don't. Normally, you don't even need scans; a skilled practitioner will be able to diagnose the cause from their assessment and start an immediate treatment plan.

Similarly, with chronic knee pain, people are often

referred for scans which show wear and tear. A doctor may conclude that the knee pain is a result of the wear and tear and start treating the knee. But how do they know that the wear and tear inside the knee is the cause of the knee pain? It could be referred pain from somewhere else in the body. Unless you also have a comparison scan, how do they know that these changes weren't there before the knee pain?

It is more effective to have a thorough assessment first and then start treatment. With chronic pain, the reality is that the treatment is unlikely to differ, regardless of what the scans and x-rays show.

WHAT THE RESEARCH TELLS US

How do you explain that when you get a typical headache, an MRI scan will show your brain is normal? How do you explain to people who didn't know they had narrowed discs in their necks because they never had neck problems?

There has been a lot of research done to prove that scans and x-rays alone can't accurately show chronic pain. In fact, at present, there are no tests to show pain.

People who had problems shown on their scans, but experienced no pain

In one study, 98 people without any back pain underwent an MRI scan. The results showed that only 36 per cent had what was considered to be a *normal* spine, while 56 per cent had bulging on at least one level and 27 per cent had a protrusion..

In another study, 67 individuals with no back pain had MRI scans done. About one-third had significant abnormality, and 35 per cent of those aged 20 to 39 years had a degenerative or bulging disc at multiple levels.

Both studies showed that you were just as likely to find

degenerative changes on a scan regardless of whether or not the subject had chronic pain. These studies clearly showed that a diagnosis such as *degenerative discs* doesn't actually mean you have an abnormal spine.

One study of computed tomography scans found that about 35 per cent of the participants who had never reported having back pain, actually had abnormalities in their spines.

In another study, 36 people with no back pain underwent MRI scans. Of these, 81 per cent had bulging discs, and 27 per cent had tears in their discs.

Remember with these studies, none of the subjects had back pain.

Given the research, in most cases, if you look at a scan of someone with chronic pain, it would probably look no different than if they didn't have chronic pain

The difference between scans and pain levels

Consider the following excerpt from a specialist's report. This report on a person who had chronic back pain stated that there was an improvement in the spine from the first MRI scan to the second.

INVESTIGATIONS:
I viewed CT scan of the lumbar sacral spine dated 2 November 2006 and two MRI scans dated at 10th April 2007 and 31st January 2008. All of them show disc pathology on the right side at L4/5. There is difference between the two MRI scans with some improvement in appearances of the disc prolapse suggesting some resorption.

The body's ability to heal over time with activity

Unfortunately for the patient, their pain had in fact gradually worsened.

What does this mean? It means that given time, your body will typically heal itself, but the pain may continue. You just need to stay healthy and active. The reality is that scans don't tell the whole story. They are just one piece of the jigsaw puzzle and a broader understanding is needed to put the pieces together and see the *whole* picture.

CHANGING OUR THINKING

It is human nature to have a negative or fearful response when we've been diagnosed with a condition. Imagine a doctor telling you that you have degenerative disc disease and that you need to, 'be careful otherwise you might end up in a wheelchair.' Now imagine if four other doctors told you that there is nothing wrong with degenerative discs. Would you ignore what that first doctor told you? Probably not. This is because your instinct is to survive and, therefore, you can't ignore the warning given by the first doctor. When these frightening descriptions and unhelpful advice are planted in your mind, it is almost impossible to dismiss your fears.

Remember your brain is designed to protect you from actual and potential danger, so your mind will always be wary of potential risks. This is just who we are. Recognise that this is normal, and challenge your unhelpful thinking. Get your doctor to explain things clearly until you understand completely. Change your mind-set.

You can see from the research that tests on people with chronic pain often come back normal.

Think of it like this. You may have had a prolapsed disc a year ago and you still have pain. You have some scans done, and the results are the same as when you had them, say six months ago. The scans show scar tissue and evidence of the prolapse. This is actually a good sign. It means that despite your persistent pain, there is no further damage. It means that your pain isn't a sign of further damage, but it is the result of over-sensitive nerves.

On the flip side, if you have chronic pain and your tests don't show anything, this is also a good thing. It means that you don't have anything structurally wrong with your body: there are no slipped discs, there are no cancers and there are no compressed nerves. It just means that your nerves are more sensitive than normal.

Remember that most people who have chronic pain report increased pain levels with changes in the weather. The weather doesn't cause more pain increase – it is just that their nerves are more sensitive.

No matter which scenario fits you best, it is difficult to accept because we all want to know what is causing the pain. Unfortunately, this is not always possible. The important thing is managing it. Managing your pain means getting on with your life and doing the things you want to do in a manageable way. Managing pain means you will feel it less. Using the strategies in this book will help enormously.

JOINT NOISES

People can be fearful of the noises that their joints make. They might stop activity because they're worried that a grating knee or grinding shoulder is a warning sign of damage. This chapter explores what the most common sounds are, and what causes them.

SNAP, CRACKLE AND POP

Sometimes our joints make funny noises: grinding, twanging, click-clacking and cracking. If we hear these noises, we can feel a little worried that they might mean there is something wrong. Conversely, most of us don't think twice about getting our backs cracked.

In general, joint noises are completely normal unless they come with extreme amounts of pain and discomfort. Below are explanations for the most common joint noises to set your mind at ease next time you make a funny sound.

THE GRINDING OR GRATING

Our knees grate and grind most in the course of performing a squatting motion. Squat down, grate, grind, stand up straight again. Sound familiar?

The tendon that attaches the kneecap to the lower leg consists of a fibrous cartilage that allows for smooth movement. This fibrous cartilage is also found behind the kneecap to help keep it in place. When you bend your knees and straighten, the fibrous cartilage rubs on the bone and other cartilage, making a grating noise. Some people may not hear it at all, while for others, it is very loud. This is completely normal, provided there is no excruciating pain.

THE CLICK-CLICK OR THE TWANG

If you rotate your wrists or ankles and made a clicking sound, or squat down and get up and your hips click, these aren't actually your joints cracking. Often, people who have been inactive and then start to exercise hear these noises and begin to worry that their joints have become weak.

Most bones have bumps and grooves on them. As you move, your tendons and ligaments flick over the bumps and grooves. A typical active person won't usually hear any noises because their tendons and ligaments are well lubricated and supple. In a less-active person, their tendons and ligaments are often drier and less supple, and when they are used, they flick over the bumps and grooves on the bones causing a click or a twang. Sometimes this may cause a bit of pain, but with stretches and exercises, your ligaments and tendons will become more lubricated, and the clicking will reduce.

Some people naturally have more lax or tight tendons and ligaments than others, and these noises are common despite their activity levels. These noises may never go away, but they are normal if there is not a lot of accompanying pain. In most cases, they are not a sign of ongoing damage.

THE CRACK

Sometimes, on TV a character will stumble around in pain and then get their back cracked to feel instant relief.

It makes you imagine that something has clicked out of place and can therefore be clicked back in. This isn't true. The immediate relief also doesn't last. Here's what really happens.

When you get your back cracked, the therapist will ask you to take a deep breath in, and then slowly breathe out and relax. As you do this, they press down and make a sudden thrusting motion with their hands and you hear a crack.

When the therapist presses down, they create a vacuum pressure in your joint, which then draws oxygen and nitrogen out of the thin film of nutritious fluid lubricating the cartilage. As these gases are drawn out, they form a bubble. This bubble then explodes into hundreds of tiny bubbles. The formation and explosion of the bubble is the crack that you hear.

When your back is cracked, a message is sent to the spinal cord, which in turn, sends instructions to muscles surrounding the joint to relax – almost like a reflex action. Afterwards, you typically feel loose and get some relief. A therapist can't crack the same joint again for about thirty minutes because it takes this long for the gases to settle back into the fluid. After a while, your muscles will tighten up again and the pain will return.

There are times when this cracking is the treatment of choice, but only for specific acute pain conditions. Using this technique for chronic pain is not as helpful, and often you risk aggravating your symptoms. Physicians are beginning to understand that regular cracking at the hands of a therapist, or even cracking your knuckles, may result in micro damage to the cartilage. Over time, this could lead to arthritis.

Some people think that cracking aligns or adjusts the spine. But logically, if the cracking gives you relief by relaxing the muscles that align or adjust your spine, then it was the tight muscles that must have amplified the pain in the first place, not your spine.

Therefore, a daily stretch and exercise program, which will help to relax muscles, is a better long-term option. Relaxed muscles mean less tension; less tension means red lights on the pain highway, and that means less pain.

FLARE-UPS AND SETBACKS

There will be times when you will experience pain levels beyond what are normal for you. Sometimes there is valid reason for this – you may have overdone things. But sometimes, because pain is unpredictable, it can flare up for no reason. Unfortunately, this is the nature of most chronic pain conditions. This chapter explores the two types of pain increases: flare-ups and setbacks.

FLARE-UPS

An increase in pain that is above normal levels and lasts a day or two, I call a *flare-up*. A flare-up doesn't mean a new injury or further damage to an old injury. It is just your nerves being more sensitive than normal. It could be because you have overdone something, have been in a stressful situation, or it could even be caused by a change in the weather. Often, with an increase in pain, you may also feel pins and needles, muscle spasms, agitation and distress.

Because most people don't really understand the nature of flare-ups, they usually increase their medication, rest in bed or even admit themselves to hospital.

Don't fall into this trap.

For chronic pain, these solutions are not solutions at all. Medication and rest, or going back for regular treatment sessions with your physiotherapist will not help in the long run; the quickest solution is not necessarily the best one.

The key to managing a flare-up is to stick to your routine. You may decide to do things a bit slower, but don't stop or avoid anything. You may also decide to use heat and ice – that is fine. Do what is needed to manage the pain, but don't avoid anything. The flare-up will pass.

By sticking to your routine, you will give yourself the confidence that your body can manage unexpected increases in pain levels. You will also understand that they are only temporary.

SETBACKS

There are times however when flare-ups last longer than just a couple of days. When this happens, I call this a *setback*. It is important to know the difference between the two, because the way you address them is different.

Setbacks are just that – they set you back a few extra days. Setbacks are often more intense than flare-ups, and like flare-ups, sometimes can occur for no obvious reason.

When you are experiencing a setback, it will be too hard to maintain your regular routine. It just won't work, even if you try to slow things down.

What you will need is a setback plan. A setback plan allows you to give your body a break. It involves cutting all your activities back by half, but then increasing your activity back to where you were within a couple of weeks. Imagine you had worked up to a daily half-hour walk. During a setback, decrease it to fifteen minutes a day, and aim to build it back up to half an hour in two to three weeks. While it seems like a backwards step, it is not.

A setback plan should only be used when things are really tough. If you use this too often, your body gets used to it and the effect is lost.

Remember, if you manage your pain well, setbacks are rare.

When some people with chronic pain experience a flare-up or setback, they become over-cautious about how they bend, how they sit, how they walk, what they do and how they do it. It is easy to get caught up in the quest to avoid flare-ups and setbacks, and not realise that they are unavoidable. It is also easy to become anxious and fearful of flare-ups, but when this happens the pain traffic lights stay green and pain worsens.

To alleviate these anxieties and fears, and to regain confidence, your thinking needs to change from wanting to avoid a flare-up, to knowing that, if you do have one, you will deal with it and manage it successfully.

A Buddhist priest, the venerable Horowpothane Sathin-driya, once said, 'Your setbacks are the pillars of your success.' He has a point; learn from your flare-ups and setbacks and you will succeed in managing your pain.

INVASIVE OPTIONS

Many chronic pain conditions have no discernible cause, yet surgery is commonly offered as a treatment option. This chapter explores common surgical options and describes the benefits and risks involved.

UNDER THE KNIFE

Surgery is really helpful in cases where there is a definite reason for a surgical solution. For example, if you have a fracture, surgery can align and pin the fracture, allowing the fracture to heal properly. Or if you have large gall-stones, surgery to remove them will help relieve the pain.

No one can use surgery to cure pain, but surgery can be used to fix the problem that might be causing the pain, but this may or may not result in pain relief. If there isn't a clear diagnosis, then surgery really isn't the answer.

As you now know, chronic pain is complex and is connected to how your nervous system works. You can only completely remove pain if you can fix the abnormal activity of the nerves. At present, there is no surgical procedure that can do that.

SPINAL SURGERY

A common type of surgery for back pain is spinal surgery. These surgeries can remove bits of bone from the spine, remove discs or fuse bones. Other surgeries involve cutting nerves in the spinal cord. People often believe that cutting a nerve will help stop the pain; unfortunately it is not that simple.

Some research suggests that four years after spinal surgery for chronic pain, patients are no better off than those who had used non-invasive strategies such as regular exercise and stretching. It is important to weigh up the options instead of rushing to the operating theatre.

INJECTIONS

Some people try injections in the hope of finding relief from pain. While they can be effective if directed at the pain source, the problem for people with chronic pain is that often there is no discernible source. Typical injections include: local anaesthetics or nerve blocks; steroid or cortisone injections; and phenol injections.

Nerve blocks can help relieve chronic pain, but in general they don't appear to have lasting effects. There have even been cases where the pain has been aggravated as a result of the injection and these patients have reported the pain as being twice as bad as it was before the injection.

Steroid or cortisone injections can provide temporary pain relief, but they are usually only used up to three times with several months in between each injection. These injections can cause bones to become brittle. Unfortunately, some of my patients tell me that they have been having cortisone shots several times a year for many years.

Phenol injections are used to destroy nerves, but at times they don't destroy all the necessary nerves and there is no guarantee of a permanent pain-free outcome. Of all the people with whom I have worked, I have only met a couple who have had permanent pain-relief as a result of phenol injections. These people saw me before having the injections and then came back afterwards for a review. Weigh this up against the risks of having phenol – which is an acid – injected into your body. You should be cautious if it is recommended to you.

Despite the risks associated with injections, they do have a role in pain management. They can offer short-term benefits. If the injection is going to help you get back on your feet and start being active, it is worthwhile discussing with your treating practitioners.

SPINAL DRUG PUMPS

Spinal-drug pumps are sometimes used in the treatment of chronic pain. They are surgically implanted beneath the skin and deliver small quantities of a drug, usually morphine, into the fluid around the spinal cord. The benefit of the pump is that it achieves the same effect by delivering only a fraction (at least 200 times less) of the drug required if given by mouth. Because less of the drug is given, there are fewer side effects. The pump has been particularly useful in some cases of cancer pain and in particular cases of spinal cord injury. However, drug pumps are only used in selective cases because they don't benefit everyone. Risks include infection, loss of menstruation in females and impotence in males. If the pump needs replacing, it requires a surgical procedure.

SPINAL CORD STIMULATORS

Another implantation device is called the spinal cord stimulator. It involves a transient electrical nerve stimulation unit being surgically implanted under the skin and connected to small electrical terminals which are surgically inserted near the spinal cord. Buzzing sensations from the spinal-cord stimulator distract the brain from concentrating on the pain. The intensity is controlled using a small hand-held remote control. However, it is not a cure and it does not work for everyone. The units alone can cost tens of thousands of dollars, in addition to the cost of surgery.

One of the big potential complications is the wires breaking inside the body and requiring further surgery to replace them. Another complication is the risk of infection. These expensive units may also require adjustments or even replacement, which means further surgery. In general, spinal cord stimulators are only effective in selected cases and long-term use may build a tolerance.

These are the invasive options available in the management of pain. These may be options for you, but regardless, the strategies outlined in this book are essential for successfully managing pain. These strategies may help you to avoid surgery, and if not, they will put you in the healthiest physical and emotional state if you do decide to have surgery.

THE ROLE OF MEDICATION

A lot of medications are taken by people with chronic pain. Some doctors are quick to prescribe painkillers, anti-inflammatory pills or cortisone shots, and patients take these simply because their doctor has prescribed them. With so many different names and families of drugs, people get confused about what they are actually taking. This chapter explores some of the more common drugs prescribed to people with chronic pain, what they actually do, and their side-effects. It also helps inform people that drugs alone are not the long-term solution.

PILLS, PILLS AND MORE PILLS

Medication can play a very important role in managing acute pain. More often than not, medication will help alleviate the pain and aid the recovery process. We've all taken an aspirin to cure a headache, or an anti-inflammatory for a rolled ankle. These medications work.

With chronic pain, medication can be used effectively to reduce pain to a manageable level and can allow you to get fitter and healthier and function on a daily basis. But with the use of medication, the focus should always be to wean off them over time. We now know that continued use of medications as the only form of pain management is not effective and that other approaches can give better results.

Most medications used in pain management aren't

actually designed to treat chronic pain, but in certain dosages, they can have pain relieving properties. These include anti-depressants, tranquillisers, anti-hypnotics, anti-convulsants, anti-epileptics and opioids. These medications are very effective in treating the conditions for which they were designed for, such as depression, schizophrenia, epilepsy and cancer, but when it comes to treating most types of chronic pain, it is a different story.

The long-term use of these medications, particularly in high doses, is not helpful in most chronic pain conditions – some of the few exceptions are cancer pain and some arthritic conditions. The long-term use of pain medication can be addictive and even fatal. Heath Ledger, Michael Jackson, Elvis Presley, Anna Nicole Smith, Brittany Murphy and Marilyn Monroe all died from overdosing on some form of pain medication.

Often prescribed by willing doctors, people may continue to take pain medications, but over time, their bodies build a tolerance to the drug and they require higher doses to have the same effect. Michael Jackson was reported to have been taking painkillers of the strength of a hospital anaesthetic. After years of regular use, his tolerance was clearly far greater than the average person's.

Generally speaking, when pain is acute, medication can be very helpful. But the aim always has to be to cut down the medication and replace it with the body's natural painkillers that kick in when activity levels increase and thinking changes for the better. Of course, in the short-term, medications may supplement the body's natural painkillers, but as the dosages increase, so do the side effects.

Some doctors may not have this understanding. They will continue to prescribe medication while not offering you alternatives such as those suggested in this book.

If you do decide to take medication long-term, you need to understand the following:

- There are no drugs at present that cure chronic pain.
- Pain medication can interfere with memory and concentration. Many people on pain medication report that their mind seems clouded.
- All medications have side effects that alter mood, energy levels, sleep, concentration and motivation.
- Pain medications can be very expensive and not give you the results you expect.
- Many people become dependent on painkillers.
- Old medications are sometimes re-packaged as new ones. If the old drug was of little benefit, the new drug may be similar.
- Stopping medications suddenly can cause with-drawal symptoms such as sleep disturbances, nausea, sweating and feelings of anxiety.

TYPES OF PAINKILLERS

Typical drug families are discussed below. Sometimes more drugs are prescribed to counteract the side effects of pain medication. If you are taking a pain medication, you can check the family to which it belongs.

NON-OPIATES

These include non-steroidal anti-inflammatory drugs (NSAIDs) such as:
- aspirin
- ibuprofen
- diclofenac.

NSAIDs reduce inflammation caused by tissue damage (for example, a sprained ankle or a bruise). Unfortunately, inflammation associated with most chronic pain conditions (unlike arthritis, nerve lesions and cancers) is due to changes in circulation, and not tissue damage. Therefore, NSAIDs are often ineffective in the treatment of chronic pain.

NSAIDs are most effective in the first ten days of an injury. Taking NSAIDs for chronic pain is unlikely to help in most cases. What these drugs will do is irritate your stomach and may cause ulcers. These drugs can also trigger asthma attacks in patients sensitive to NSAIDs. In extreme cases of patients who have other medical complications, NSAIDs can also trigger heart failure and renal failure.

OPIATES

The most common opiates prescribed for pain are:
- codeine
- dihydrocodeine
- morphine
- tramadol (weak opioid)
- dextropropoxyphene.

Opiates work by blocking pain messages both at the site of the injury and in the brain. While these drugs might be helpful in the short-term, in the long-term, they have significant side effects, often causing changes in mood, drowsiness, headaches, nausea, constipation, and difficulties with concentration and memory.

Ironically, to counter these side effects, doctors often prescribe more medication.

Over time, your body becomes tolerant to opiates and you start to gradually increase the dose; this is called dependency. Unfortunately, higher doses only result in stronger unwanted side effects, not a reduction of your pain. The latest research suggests that instead of being a painkiller, opiate-based drugs can act as pain amplifiers.

ANTI-DEPRESSANTS

There are many different types of anti-depressants. Some of the more common anti-depressants are:
- amitriptyline
- nortriptyline
- doxepin
- trimipramine
- fluoxetine
- sertraline
- fluvoxamine
- mirtazapine
- venlafaxine
- duloxetine.

Anti-depressants are prescribed for several reasons in the treatment of pain. In higher doses, they lift your mood, in lower doses, they act as a painkiller. Side effects include: drowsiness, weight gain, constipation, blurred vision, dry mouth, dizziness, difficulty urinating, poor concentration and clouded judgement. Mixed with alcohol, anti-depressants can be fatal.

SEDATIVES OR TRANQUILLISERS

Sedatives or tranquillisers are often given as a short-term treatment to help you sleep, or calm you down. Common forms are:
- barbiturates (amobarbital, pentobarbital)
- benzodiazepines (diazepam, flunitrapezam, alprazolam, temazepam)
- herbal sedatives (marijuana, katnip)
- solvent sedatives (diethyl ether, methyl trichloride)
- non-benzodiazepines (zopiclone, zolpidem)
- antidepressants (mirtazapine, trazodone)

- antipsychotics (haloperidol, fluphenazine, clozapine, olanzapine)
- opiates (morphine, codeine)

Sedatives act on the central nervous system to relax muscles and help you sleep. Side effects include: slurred speech, staggering gait, poor judgement, tiredness to the point of passing out, depression and disturbed sleep patterns.

ANTI-CONVULSANTS

Anti-convulsants were originally designed to treat epilepsy. However, today they are also used in the treatment of chronic pain. Some of the most common anti-convulsants are:

- gabapentin
- pregabalin
- carbamazapine
- sodium valproate

Anti-convulsants are thought to act on the brain and the central nervous system to diminish pain messages. Unfortunately, the body usually builds a tolerance to them. Strong side effects include: extreme sleepiness and tiredness; dizziness and headaches; weight gain; stomach upsets; forgetfulness and shakiness.

STEROIDS

Steroids are frequently used in chronic conditions, such as rheumatoid arthritis, to reduce inflammation. In chronic pain, they can be given into the joints by injections, such as cortisone injections. Prolonged use has shown to increase the risk of osteoporosis, weight gain, diabetes and depression.

LOCAL ANAESTHETICS

Local anaesthetics act on nerves and the spinal cord to block pain messages. They are administered by injection. These drugs often relieve pain but leave an area of numbness or muscle weakness. In most chronic pain cases, they are not recommended for long-term use.

As you can see, there are many medications on the market to treat chronic pain. While these may have their benefits, the alternative methods in this book are more sustainable in the long-term than most drug treatments. Importantly, a combination of stretching, gentle exercise, pacing, and a positive mindset don't come with side effects.

I have had first-hand experience of these side effects. When I was stuck in hospital for five weeks following my collapsed lung, I was given strong painkillers four times a day for five weeks. I felt dazed and confused, and I became so constipated that my bowels and bladder stopped working properly. I then had to endure the humiliation of being given a suppository. With my burns, the medications not only made me feel jet-lagged and constipated but they also gave me cold sweats. And to think, I only took medication for a relatively short period compared with some of my clients. I can only imagine their struggle.

If you are not managing your pain, or have been using medications for a long time, discuss a medication reduction plan with your doctor. Then, as you decrease your dosage, use the strategies taught in this book as a replacement for the reduction in dosage.

A final caution: if you are on medications, you should never stop taking them suddenly. See your doctor to discuss and formulate a medication reduction plan.

RELATIONSHIPS AND INTIMACY

Most people with chronic pain have concerns about intimacy at some point, but finding answers can be embarrassing or difficult. This chapter explores ways to plan and prepare for intimate situations so that people with chronic pain can feel more confident.

THE FEAR FACTOR

For someone with chronic pain, intimacy is often an awkward topic of discussion, but can be a very real issue. It is common to hear statements like:

- I'm just too scared to get into a relationship. What if my pain stops me from satisfying my partner?
- What if I get stuck in a position? What if I make my partner feel guilty if I end up in pain?
- Trying to explain it to them might put them off.
- It's just too hard. There are more important things to do.

But of course, intimacy is important. Sharing happiness and being in love are precious. We can show our love in many ways: a warm hug, a cuddle or when we make love.

The fear of disappointing yourself and others during intimacy is a major concern to people in pain. Another fear is that intimate relations will lead to more pain. Such anxieties are often compounded by partners, as they worry about causing more pain to their loved one.

Many pain sufferers avoid intimacy or don't actively seek out relationships. In their eyes, it's safer to stay single or avoid intimacy.

Despite Hollywood movies showing us that passion is about spontaneity, immediacy and acrobatics, the reality is that sex does not have to be spontaneous for it to be good. It is something that can be planned for.

PLANNING FOR INTIMACY

It is important to talk about this sensitive topic with your partner. Speaking openly and sharing your thoughts and anxieties may help in the long term and address any assumptions you both may have. You can use the same strategies that you use for your pain to help improve your intimate relations. Initially, it may feel structured but this will help you get started.

Set goals

Remember, goals need to be realistic and achievable. If you are already in a relationship, think of goals that may help improve your intimacy – perhaps going away for a weekend or going for a romantic dinner. If you are not in a relationship but would like to be, set a goal to go out and meet people.

Preparing

Completing your stretches and exercises regularly will give you fitness and flexibility for intimacy.

Challenging unhelpful thoughts

We know that our thoughts affect how we feel. If you are having negative thoughts about intimacy because of your pain, challenge them and don't assume the worst.

Relaxation techniques

It may help to practice some relaxation techniques before and after any sexual activity. Try to relax together so that a better understanding is established. Some people find gentle massage helpful for each other to relax before, during and afterwards. Ambiance using candles or incense is another way to create a serene and relaxed atmosphere.

PRACTICAL INTIMACY

Pain clinics all over the world suggest many different processes to their patients to help initiate intimacy. There are no set rules about how to become more intimate. Here is one example:

Improving your sexual relationship

Pick a time where you will not be interrupted or rushed. Wear clothing that may arouse your partner. You need to feel comfortable but sexually appealing to your partner. Come to the understanding that there will be no penetrative sex for three to four weeks. This will help ease any anxieties about performance, and it is a reminder that this process is there to help create an atmosphere and assist with your intimacy. It is recommended that this process be done two or three times per week.

Step 1
- Ensure that your partner is lying face down. This will give you a sense of control and also some comfort that you are not being watched.
- Relax your partner in their desired way, for example, give them a massage. Stroke the length of their body except their genitals.
- Encourage them to participate by asking them to direct your hands and tell you what they would like you to do.
- Change roles after about ten minutes, and ensure that you find a comfortable position.
- Complete this step for a week or two, or until both of you feel completely comfortable.

Step 2
- Do as before, but now also explore the genital areas
- Get your partner lying on their back and explore their whole body including the genitals. The idea is to give you confidence to know that you are allowing them to watch what you are doing.
- Ask them what is pleasurable.
- Change positions.
- Remember, no penetrative sex.
- Complete this step for at least two weeks, or until both of you feel completely comfortable.

Step 3
- Now, you may have penetrative sex, but it is best if is not demanded.
- Incorporate penetrative sex, but ensure that you focus on your own desires, with your partner being the passive one.
- Swap roles once you feel comfortable.
- Explore positions and activities that are comfortable for you.

HAVING FUN

Some of the most frequent questions about intimate practices are about pacing. Here are some typical questions:

- How am I going to pace myself?
- I can only be on my back for a couple of minutes. How can I stop and ask to change positions?
- How do I stop my back from cramping up?

Pacing is important. Some pain sufferers use songs as timers. When the song changes, so does their position. A typical song is a couple of minutes long so change positions with the change of songs. Be creative. Talk to your partner. Some people might even have a clock in their line of sight to have a quick glance.

There is a saying: *We come to love not by finding a perfect person, but by learning to see an imperfect person perfectly.* Whoever said that was spot on.

TO WORK OR NOT TO WORK

If you are a working age but have stopped working because of your pain, this section is very important for you. In my experience, some doctors just don't seem to understand the importance of their patients returning to work after an injury. Often, returning to work is seen as something that comes after the treatments have finished, or when the pain has been cured. This chapter explores the vital importance of work as a part of rehabilitation.

THE ROLE OF WORK

Work is not just about earning money. It is about much more. Work gives you self-worth. It gives you an opportunity to succeed and advance. It comes with a social outlet. You get to leave the house. Work helps you buy a house. Work is separate from your family and gives you the chance to shine outside your family. Work gives you status. Work gives you a routine.

Work is about so much more than just money.

It's hard for people if their pain stops them from working. Think about it. All of a sudden your routine is broken. Your financial independence might be lost, along with your status within your family and social circles.

But it's not just about you either.

Recent research into the effect of parental unemployment on children has found that the children are more likely to grow and be out of work themselves, either for periods of time or entirely. This research also found that they were also more susceptible to psychological distress resulting in withdrawal, anxiety and depression, or aggressive behaviour, including substance abuse. They are also more likely to experience chronic pain.

So no, it's not just about you; it can affect your kids too.

Being off work can affect your sleep patterns as well. You don't use your energy in the way that you did when you worked. As a result, you won't sleep as well because your energy levels haven't been drained like they are when you work. You can become bored and lethargic, and of course, you have more time to focus on your pain than you would if you were working. People who come to my clinic often say that they feel as though they are jet-lagged. Their body clock is shot; they sleep during the day, and can't sleep at night. *Jet-lagged* is a really good description. You may relate to this. You also may relate to the fact that a flurry of medical appointments can quickly replace work. This lethargy and boredom and focusing on pain leads to a negative state of mind and the traffic lights on the pain highway remain green.

However much people try to convince themselves that prolonged rest eases their pain, the research does not support this. In the time I have been doing this work, I have *never* met a chronic pain sufferer who felt better after staying at home for lengthy periods.

Another important thing to consider is that research has shown that the longer a person with chronic pain is off work, the harder it is for them to return. In fact, after around three months of being off work, the likelihood of ever returning to any work drops to around 50 per cent.

But don't worry; it's never too late to go back.

In one study, 72 people who returned to work as part

of their pain rehabilitation reported increased levels of activity and at the same time, significant reductions in their pain. The study listed the many benefits of returning to work.

Also, recent reviews from the United Kingdom that investigated whether work is good for your health and well-being concluded that overall, the benefits of working outweighed the risks. It also showed that the health benefits of working were much greater than the harmful effects of long-term unemployment or prolonged sickness absence.

To help encourage people with pain to return to work, the attitudes of some health practitioners need to be challenged. One of the biggest barriers to returning to work is the failure of health practitioners to recognise its importance. Often, they won't even discuss it. Many of my clients have told me how their doctors have told them not to even entertain the thought of returning to work until they have been cured of their pain. Unfortunately, this advice adds to the vicious cycle of suffering.

A recent study conducted in the Netherlands highlighted this very point. That study interviewed 252 injured workers. It found an overall lack of discussion by doctors and specialists about returning to work, and concluded that, if a greater focus was put on returning to work, there would have been better outcomes for those injured workers.

What the experts say...

A recent document developed by the Australasian Faculty of Occupational and Environmental Medicine reviewed literature on the health benefits of work and concluded that work was good for health and wellbeing. It said that extended time off work resulted in a worsening of symptoms rather than improving them.

It reported that being off work for a long time:

- increased the rates of mortality for cardiovascular diseases and suicide
- had far worse risks than some of the most dangerous jobs
- resulted in poorer general health
- resulted in poorer physical and psychological health
- had a negative impact on families

This document was endorsed by many international professional bodies including the internationally renowned Royal Australian College of Physicians and the Royal Australian College of General Practitioners.

This kind of document packs a punch. Higher risk of heart and lung problems, suicide, poor general health, poor physical and psychological health... it is a grim picture. Contrast this with the benefits of work, and you will clearly see that work and activity are the solutions.

Being at work, in any capacity, will give you a sense of self-worth as well as improve your concentration, social circles, family dynamics, sleep, and fitness. It will also help you to manage your pain much better.

Returning to work is a part of returning to life.

NO WIN, NO FEE: WHAT IT REALLY COSTS YOU

We've all heard the ads on the radio and TV that tell us if we are injured at work there are legal firms who will work on a no win, no fee basis. They market the idea really well – they will take your case on and your employer to court if needed and get you a big pay-out and then you can all live happily ever after. It's the happily ever after bit that most people don't think about.

If you injure yourself at work, you deserve the right advice and to be compensated. But it doesn't always happen this way.

Here's an example of advice that looked good at the time, but in the long-term was quite damaging. Max was a 40-year-old truck driver at a big transport company. One day, his foot slipped as he was climbing out of his truck cabin and he landed heavily on his right knee, damaging the cartilage. His employer was supportive and paid for the arthroscope and rehabilitation he needed afterwards. On advice, Max found a lawyer who could get him a payout.

Unfortunately for Max, his lawyer was all about the money, but that kind of approach wasn't helpful to him. Throughout his legal proceedings, Max was sent to a number of different specialists, who all confirmed that he had sustained an injury that may prevent him from driving trucks.

While Max was suffering with his bad knee, a part of him was a bit excited at the notion of a payout. The lawyer had talked in the tens of thousands of dollars – or even higher if he was judged to have a permanent disability that stopped him from driving trucks again. He felt justified in his claim because every day, his knee seemed to feel worse. As he went for test after test, he repeated his story to each doctor. Because his life was now largely focused on his injury and the doctors and lawyers, his conversations with his friends and family became about his pain, his case, and he said with a sigh at the end of every conversation, 'I'll probably never drive a truck again.' His mindset had become very negative.

Max then came to my clinic and I suggested returning to work in a limited capacity to help him get back to his normal routine. Max was keen to try it until he told his lawyers. They explained to him that going back to work may affect his payout. Max stopped coming. I was told by his wife that he had found a new therapist who told him not to consider returning to work before signing up for fifty therapy treatments.

After four long years of tests and court hearings – which he had not realised was the average for these types of cases – Max was diagnosed with a permanent disability and was thrilled when the court finally awarded him a higher sum than he had expected. He returned home with his portion of the payout (after paying his legal fees and other costs) to live the happily ever after ending that he had imagined.

Only that didn't happen.

Max paid off his mortgage, which made him and his wife very happy, but then he had very little left of his payout. He had been deemed unfit for work and Max agreed with the court's decision. He felt unfit, lethargic, depressed and useless. Every day, Max said goodbye to his wife as she dressed and left for the office. Every evening, she returned home full of stories about her day, her challenges and triumphs. Some nights, she didn't get home until late because she would go out for work drinks. Max never wanted to join her because the one time he did go, he had nothing to say. He had tried explaining about his pain and his compensation payout, but people soon looked bored and left to talk to someone else.

The disability pension which looked okay at the time,

soon proved inadequate. More and more, Max relied on his wife to make up the shortfall in the family's financial accounts. More and more, he felt useless.

Max often remembered the advice I had given him about the gradual return to work. All things considered, he wished that he had at least given it a try. Looking back, he realised that for the five years following the knee injury, he had undergone almost every test known to man, but hadn't really been encouraged by his doctors or his lawyers to seek effective treatments that might help.

Long after the compensation ran out, Max still had to live his life and pay his bills. For Max, there was no happily ever after. But it didn't have to be this way; getting a lesser payout, and returning to some work, could have allowed Max to earn more, and become financially wealthier in the long term. Not just that, but he would be healthier and happier for it. Luckily for Max, he came back to my clinic, and I was able to help him.

There are numerous studies on the effect of litigation on chronic pain, and almost all conclude that litigation tends to increase pain levels. One study involving 200 chronic pain participants measured pain levels, disability and depression. The study found that the participants who were working and not seeking compensation were less depressed, less debilitated and in less pain than people who were not working and were in the process of litigation. Another study of 484 adults with chronic pain found that litigation for chronic pain was strongly associated with higher levels of pain-related disability.

So the legal process that compensates you for your pain can at times actually *cause* you more pain.

It's better to use the right legal advice to get the necessary compensation, and while you're doing that, return to work.

And you're not on your own. Most developed countries also have compensation schemes to support people injured at work. These schemes work exceptionally well and are very beneficial when used correctly. The most effective way to use these schemes is to get the funding for the right treatment, and if it is safe to do so, try and return to work while you have that treatment. These schemes may also be used as a financial top-up, or used to help you find more suitable work. Essentially, focusing on returning to work with use of these schemes and the right advice is best.

If you can't find something at your own workplace that suits your abilities, then try to find another job, or do some volunteer work until you can return. Remember, it's not just about the money, it's about self-worth, independence, quality of life and socialising – none of which can ever be compensated properly with money. Remember also that a return to work is a part of returning to life.

Of course, there are exceptions where some people are unable to work due to the severity of their injuries. But this is only a very small group.

A SUCCESSFUL RETURN

The first step to a successful return to work is that you have to *want* to work. You need to feel in control of your rehabilitation and you need to plan to overcome any obstacles. Returning to work is not just about you; you are not on your own. You need to involve other people: your employer, your co-workers, your doctors, your family and any other services that are there to support you. Often, having a meeting with everyone allows you to put any issues and concerns on the table and find solutions and common goals. If everyone is informed, there won't be any surprises, and everyone will understand their roles. In cases where there was a significant injury, it is unrealistic to expect an injured worker to return to their pre-injury role straight away. A graded return to work is necessary, and has been demonstrated to be the most effective strategy. A plan outlining suitable duties and hours, timeframes and a gradual progression of duties and hours to a pre-injury level is needed.

If you have stopped working because of your pain, it may be worthwhile considering the following:

- Staying in touch with your employer and work mates.
- Having a positive attitude towards returning to work. Remember, aside from the physical and psychological benefits, it is beneficial financially, medically and socially.
- Suggesting a meeting with you, your employer and your doctor to set some return to work goals and discuss work options.

Questions for you to also consider:

- What duties do you think you can manage?
- What concerns do you have about returning to work? How can you address these?
- How are you going to get to work?
- What are your standing and sitting tolerances?
- How will you pace yourself at work?
- What strategies can you use before, during and after your shift for you to manage your symptoms?

Questions for your employer to consider:

- What suitable duties are available?
- How flexible can the working hours be?
- If no suitable duties are available, is there work at another location?

Questions for your doctor to consider:
- What can you do functionally (e.g. sitting, standing and lifting tolerances)?
- Given the health benefits of work, when can you return to work?
- If you are not ready, what further treatment, if any, do you need to allow you to become ready for work?
- Given your injury/condition, how important is incorporating a return to work into your rehabilitation?

GOALS	By (Date)	By Whom Tick (✓) appropriate			
Short term		Worker	Employer	GP/THP	Other
ABCD Manufacturing to investigate suitable duties and propose a graded return to work program	14th March				
Commence a graded return to work	21st March	✓			
Mr Black to meet with GP and endorse the return to work program	14th March	✓		✓	
Medium Term					
Progress to 50% pre-injury hours	1st May	✓			
Prepare for a trial of pre-injury duties three days per week	1st May		✓		
Meeting to review progress with all parties	8th May	✓	✓	✓	
Long Term					
Achieve a return to his pre-injury duties and hours	1st June	✓			
Mr Black's GP to clear Mr Black to return to his pre-injury position	24th May	✓		✓	
Final meeting with all parties	1st June	✓	✓	✓	

If you are of a working-age, returning to work is a key component of your rehabilitation. It is not something to consider *after* rehabilitation. Effective pain management is about getting your life back on track. Work is a part of life. Its importance should not be underestimated – just look at the research.

ERGONOMICS AND POSTURE

Plenty of pieces of furniture and equipment make claim to be ergonomic. What does this really mean? This chapter explains the key principles of ergonomics, posture and manual handling.

ERGONOMIC DESIGN

Ergonomic equipment has developed at a rapid rate. The telephone handset has become a wireless headset, there are monitor stands placed on height-adjustable desks, and of course, many of us sit on fully-adjustable tilting office chairs. Undoubtedly, ergonomic equipment has played a significant role in improving comfort, preventing injuries and assisting people get back to work and their day-to-day activities following an injury.

While there are benefits of using ergonomic equipment, the truth is that ergonomic designs are often based on the designer's understanding of ideal postures. Perfect angles are calculated, but this is where ergonomic equipment has its limits. Humans don't sit at perfect angles.

Now, there is a growing realisation of this. We simply can't cater for everyone with one piece of ergonomic equipment. Because of this, over the years, you will have noticed that the number and nature of ergonomic equipment has changed. An example is ergonomic chairs and desks: they now have more adjustment handles and more choice than ever before.

The reality is that everyone is different, and so the best thing to do is to try before you buy, and get the *right* advice.

GOOD POSTURE

We have all heard about the importance of good posture. So what is a good posture? Well, it really depends on what you are doing. While you are typing at the computer, sitting upright is ergonomically suitable and comfortable for a period of time. When watching TV on the couch, most people find it much more comfortable to recline than sit upright.

Most people have also seen health and safety diagrams at work showing figures sitting in upright positions. These figures look rigid, and not only that, those positions can't be sustained. They give general advice because, theoretically, they are ergonomic. They may be ergonomic but they are not suggesting that you adopt the postures for a long period of time. Here's why.

Good posture is any posture that is comfortable, but not sustained for a long period. Posture is not about being in a static position which gradually becomes really uncomfortable. We have all heard of bedsores suffered by people with restricted movement, or we may have experienced stiffness in our backs if we've had to sit or stand for too long. Our circulation works best when we are moving. Movement comes naturally to us. When we move – even if it is just shifting positions at our desk – the body releases a nutrient-rich fluid into our joints which helps keep them lubricated and healthy.

So choose positions that are comfortable and change positions regularly – a rule of thumb is to change position at least every twenty minutes. This is good for your joints and your circulation. It really is a case of: the best position is the next position.

For some people, ergonomic mouse pads, chairs and keyboards can be a bit of a trap because they are so comfortable. Think about it. If it is healthy to move around and change positions every twenty minutes or so, more ergonomic office equipment can lull you into a comfort zone so that you forget to move around. Ergonomic equipment is designed to make you comfortable, but use them for short periods of time.

Another piece of equipment which I see a lot in return-to-work cases is a long-handled pick-up tool prescribed for people with back injuries. Instead of bending over to pick something up, the person picks it up with the aid of this tool. In the beginning, this pick-up tool is helpful, but when you are ready, it is important to begin to bend over to pick up light objects. Make it an exercise, rather than continue to use the tool for everything and become reliant on it.

Normally, to pick something up, you use all the little muscles in your hand, arm and back in a synchronised way. By practising picking things up without equipment, you help to re-synchronise the muscle activity to allow for smoother movements. Equipment can sometimes stop you from doing this and seeing the bigger, more important picture.

SPLINTS AND BRACES

Like ergonomic equipment, splints and braces work best when they aid the rehabilitation process. A wrist splint can be used to help maintain a natural wrist posture following surgery, or in conditions involving nerve damage. A neck brace can be used to protect the spinal cord, or a knee brace to minimise movement following a knee reconstruction.

Unfortunately, some therapists are quick to prescribe splints and braces for common chronic pain conditions. The over-prescription of back braces for low back pain is a good example of this. People with back pain are often told to wear a brace when they work, when they go to the gym, and in some cases, all day long. Often, they are told that the brace will encourage good posture. Using the brace for short periods of time, when the pain is really bad, may help, but regular use of back braces for back pain is not good for you. The back brace hugs the back and gives it support, but by doing so, does what the back muscles are meant to do. Over time, by using a back brace, your back muscles are used less and hence become de-conditioned, putting your back at risk of injury.

Also, restricting movement for long periods using splints and braces can actually make the pain worse. Remember, movement can be used as a distraction from the pain, and it keeps the muscles, ligaments and joints healthy. For most chronic pain conditions, the frequent use of splints and braces is not an answer.

LIFTING SAFELY

How should you lift? When lifting something, particularly off the floor, most people have been taught that they should bend their knees and keep their backs straight. This may be good when lifting a 20 kg box, but does it make sense to use this same technique to lift a pen?

Remember that your body is designed to move in many directions. What is helpful is to assess the task and then make a conscious decision about which posture to adopt. If you keep your back straight and bend your knees every time you pick up something from the floor, you can actually increase the risk of back injury. While this may be the safest way to lift heavier objects because it uses the large leg muscles, if you do that for everything you pick up – a dropped pen, a newspaper – you won't be using the smaller muscles along your spine. If you don't use them, they will weaken, increasing the risk of injury. Remember the phrase, *use it or lose it* – there is truth in this.

If you have to lift something, remember the simple TILE principle:

T = Task
I = Individual
L= Load
E = Environment

- Task: What needs to be lifted or moved, and where does it need to go?
- Individual: Can you do it on your own or do you need assistance?
- Load: What is the size and shape of the load? How heavy is it?
- Environment: Are there any obstacles? Is the floor slippery? Is the environment safe?

Here is an example of a person using the TILE method to assess a lifting situation. Chris has to lift a 10 kg box from the floor of his office onto a chest-high shelf. He has back pain and uses the TILE method every time he lifts heavier objects. Here is how he goes through the process automatically in his head:

T = The task is to lift a 10 kg box from the floor and onto a shelf.
I = Am I able to lift the 10 kg box and put it on the shelf? Do I need help?
L = It is 10 kg. The box is a regular-shaped box. Do I need to nudge it to see?
E = Is the environment safe? Is there anything in the way?

Is the floor slippery? Does anything need to be cleared to make room before I lift the box? Are others at risk?

Ten kilograms is not an especially easy weight for him since his back problems started. He gives the box a nudge with his foot to confirm its approximate weight. He decides that, while it is heavy, it is a weight that he can manage safely. He bends his knees, securely grasps the box close to his body, straightens his legs and lifts the box. He puts it on the shelf.

As he picks up the box, Chris's pen slides out of his pocket and falls to the floor. When the box is safely on the shelf, Chris quickly goes through the TILE process again. The task this time is only picking up a pen. He knows he doesn't need to use his big leg muscles, but he also knows that he can get shooting back pain if he bends too quickly. Chris places one hand on the shelf to support himself and bends over to retrieve his pen.

In most cases, people do this automatically. However, people with chronic pain can become so focused on both their pain and the risk of re-injury that they become fearful and avoid bending altogether.

There is no doubt that ergonomic equipment is here to stay, but the important thing to remember is that good posture involves a regular change in position, irrespective of the ergonomic equipment used and how comfortable it may be. And when it comes to lifting, remember to assess the task first and work towards the normal way of doing it.

COMMUNICATION TECHNIQUES

People suffering chronic pain can find communicating about their pain very difficult. The challenge is to find the balance between explaining it so that people can support you, and going into too much detail so that people start to avoid you. This chapter explores effective ways of getting your message across to others.

A WORLD OF PAIN

Writers talk a lot about books and writing because that is their world. The conversation of an actor will be predominantly about acting and theatre, TV and movies because these things are a big part of their world. People in pain will often talk a lot about their pain because it is such a big part of their lives. But often, they feel that no one understands or that no one wants to listen. Some people with chronic pain say that they have difficulty talking about their pain to others because their pain is invisible; there is no plaster cast or sling that signifies pain. And worse for them is that x-rays and tests might not show the cause, making it even more invisible.

But let's face it; people are drawn to others who are positive, interesting and fun to be around. People are also drawn to inspirational battlers. While a monologue about your bad back may be interesting to you because it is such a huge part of your life, other people might not find it at all interesting. Therapists hear a common complaint from clients. It goes something like this: *people don't call me anymore because all I talk about is my pain and I don't do anything that is interesting to talk about.*

The opposite can occur too. Sufferers of chronic pain may not want to talk to others because they think that they have nothing to talk about besides their suffering. The pain sufferer might not want to be labelled a whinger. All of this adds to the isolation experienced by so many pain sufferers.

Then there is the person who is angry and demanding. They know best and don't want to listen to others. Everything has to be done to their expectations and time frames; there is no compromise. They might lose their temper easily and lash out.

The trick is to find the happy medium – a style of communication that clearly and politely lets people know how you're feeling, how they can help you, or if you are able to do something yourself and would rather be left to your own devices. This is called assertive communication.

BEING ASSERTIVE

Developing assertive communication skills will ensure that you have the best chance of making your thoughts and feelings known to others, and having a positive result come from this.

Characteristics of assertive communication include:
- saying things in a calm and clear way
- genuinely listening to what people say
- calmly asking people for what you want
- talking things through
- asking for other people's opinions: *what are your thoughts on this?*
- finding a way around the problem

- making 'I' statements – *I would like...*, or *I prefer ...*, instead of *you should...*
- making 'you could' statements – *you could help...*, or *you could stop...* instead of *you should...*
- allow yourself to express your feelings in an open and honest way by making statements like: *I feel nervous saying this to you but...*, or *I don't mean to offend you, but it would help if you could...*

Whenever a client comes into my clinic and describes how people aren't interested in listening when they talk about their pain, I always get them to put themselves in the listener's shoes.

How much would you want to hear about a person's pain? Never was this better illustrated than when a woman suffering chronic pain came into my clinic with her pain journal. She carried this small exercise book everywhere with her. In the journal, she had written extensively about her pain, recorded her every feeling and included coloured diagrams to indicate her pain levels at different times of the day. The entries detailed all her problems and negative feelings. She told me proudly that if someone asked her about her pain, she handed them the book so that they could read all about it. Her reasoning was that she was sick of explaining her pain story to people and the journal saved her the bother.

I acknowledged the difficulties that she was clearly facing on a daily basis. Then, as gently as possible, I asked her how she would react if someone handed their pain journal to her.

The woman looked at me without speaking. It took several moments during which I could see the slow dawning of understanding.

'I guess I probably wouldn't read all of it,' she said finally.

'So if you were making a caring enquiry about a friend's health, how much would you like them to tell you?' I asked.

'The short version.'

In that moment, I could tell she got it. All it took was to ask her to imagine herself as the listener rather than the talker.

THE SHORT VERSION

The woman got it right when she identified that people preferred the short version. The simple social greeting, 'how are you?' does not warrant anything more than a simple response. Remember, you are being asked how you are not necessarily how *your pain* is. So if need be, let them know how you are and include a pain update if things have changed, for better or worse, but remember to focus on other aspects of your life as well. Alternatively, a simple positively phrased response is even better. Try saying something such as: *I'm doing okay today or I've had some really good days lately.*

THE LONGER VERSION

Sometimes you do need to explain your pain, especially when it involves your safety or wellbeing. Just say you start a new job and you need your colleagues to understand that you might have certain limitations when it came to lifting or needing to take regular breaks. As a health and safety issue, your colleagues need to know the best way to react if your pain flares up. Do they call an ambulance? Or do they let you manage it yourself and allow you to call the shots?

To do this, focus on telling exactly what they need to know, without too much detail. Ask yourself: *If I was in their shoes, what would I want to know?* You might want to know:

- where is the pain?
- what things tend to make the pain worse?
- what helps to manage the pain?
- what can I do to help?

It is most effective if you can be the one to tell staff as a group, rather than have your supervisor pass on the information. If you tell everyone yourself, you know how much they know. You can also answer any questions they might have. The benefit here is that you only need to say it once, rather than repeat it over and over.

It can be daunting. I remember standing in front of my colleagues after I returned to Australia. My wounds had healed and I looked completely normal. I wanted them to know that, if I left my computer every half-hour to have a short break, I had to do that to manage my pain. I needed them to understand that I was still capable of doing the work, but me doing the work might look a little different to them doing the same work. This was the best way to get the message across. Speaking to my colleagues gave me a real sense of control.

Rather than describe how bad the pain is and how it negatively affects your life, focus mainly on how you manage the pain, and any ways that they can help you manage it in the workplace. People will be more willing to help you, if they can see that you are trying to help yourself.

GETTING THE MESSAGE ACROSS

A lot of pain sufferers experience frustration in their communications. A common problem is that others overcompensate or try too hard to help the sufferer, often with the best of intentions.

One woman who suffered chronic pain described how a colleague would get to the office car park early and sit in his car and wait till she arrived so that he could offer to carry her bag up several flights of stairs. There was nothing but genuine concern for the woman and she was appreciative, but this soon got annoying for her. While there were lots of things her condition prevented her from doing, she could carry her own small bag up the stairs. The problem is that, because her co-worker's act stemmed from kindness, she found it really hard to tell him she didn't need his assistance.

Instead of allowing the co-worker to continue with this, she could use any of the following responses:

- I really appreciate your help, but you can help me more by...
- Thanks for offering to carry my bag, but it's important to keep my muscle strength up and I'm trying to do it myself.
- I can manage my bag, but perhaps you can help me later with...

The opposite of the overly-helpful colleague is the unhelpful one. It is not always obvious when someone is suffering pain. This invisibility can mean that co-workers can forget or simply be too busy to notice and offer assistance. Assertive communication means that the pain sufferer needs to be polite, clear and concise when they need help or special consideration. Don't wait for others to notice. People are busy and your pain will not be at the forefront of their minds.

If you're having an increased pain day, don't be afraid to simply explain this to your colleagues. Sentences like the ones below can be a guide:

- I'm having a bad day and I would appreciate your help with...
- I'm finding this hard today, could you please...
- My back is playing up. I will only be able to stand for

short periods. Could I sit and finish some paperwork instead?

- If you could help me lift these boxes, then I can unpack them...

People are usually generous and happy to help. They are usually happy to help someone who they can see is helping themself, as opposed to someone who blames their pain and avoids activity all the time. When you get help, always remember to show your appreciation. A simple thank you is a very powerful thing.

A SERIOUS LOOK AT LAUGHTER

Laughter is therapeutic. People feel better after a good laugh. This chapter explores why this is so and shows the benefits of seeing the funny side to life, even when life doesn't seem very funny.

IS LAUGHTER REALLY THE BEST MEDICINE?

When someone is in pain, laughing might not be something they do very often. Mostly, it is because they see the world as being full of pain and suffering. Sometimes, people with pain will avoid laughter because they think that if they laugh, people won't believe they are in pain. Sometimes, people get so down that being unhappy, depressed and miserable becomes their persona.

It doesn't need to be like that. From all that we have covered so far, we know that the better our mood, the less our pain. I know this from my own experience. When I was lying in hospital with my burns, I knew right from the start that to consider what might have been, or to feel sorry for myself, would most likely lead to depression. I'm neither a glass-half-empty nor a glass-half-full kind of person. I just see the water level at half-way. For me, this was all about choosing to look on the bright side, or in my case the funny side. I think it all began when I got wrapped in cling-wrap in the emergency department to stop air getting to my burns. I could have looked at this process in horror, but instead, I said to the medical staff that I felt like I was in a giant condom. The medical staff laughed. They would never have laughed at a burns victim if I hadn't started it, but it broke the ice.

Another benefit to me joking about my situation was that the medical staff, after the laughing, seemed to want to do more for me. Even in the emergency room, the staff responded to my humour. I guess that if they spend their working days surrounded by the seriously injured or people hurt and moaning, a bit of humour stands out like a beacon.

When you are sharing a funny moment, it's almost impossible to laugh and focus on your pain at the same time.

Facts about laughter...

- Neurologist Henri Rubenstein found that one minute of solid laughter provides up to 45 minutes of subsequent relaxation.
- William Fry at Stanford University reported that 100 laughs provide your body an aerobic workout equal to that of a 10 minute session on a rowing machine.
- Laughter stimulates the body's natural painkillers and mood lifters. These have a similar chemical composition to morphine and heroin, and have a relaxing effect on the body while building up the immune system.
- Laughter increases the amount of oxygen in the blood, improves circulation and thus helps heal damaged tissues.
- Laughter helps to stimulate your appetite and burns up calories.
- Author and editor Norman Cousins (1915–1990) who published the book Anatomy of an Illness was diagnosed with ankylosing spondylitis (a potentially crippling spinal condition) and given a few months to live. In 1965, he checked himself out of hospital and into a hotel room. He exposed himself to high doses of vitamin C, watched comedies on TV and read funny books. He laughed as much as he could. His symptoms steadily decreased until he was well again. He lived for another 25 years. This remarkable story shows just how powerful laughter can be.

It is important for you to find ways to laugh more. If you feel that you don't laugh enough, consider being around people you find humorous, watch funny movies and TV shows, and attend comedy shows. Laughter releases the body's natural painkillers which will help turn the pain traffic lights to red.

Things can get really tough, but laughter can help. Even if things are overwhelming, it is okay to have a laugh. Sometimes chronic pain makes you feel isolated and as if no one understands. Sometimes, you may feel as if your whole world is about pain and everyone else's lives seem removed from yours. Laughter can be the common ground, the thing that unites people. Having a few laughs with friends and family can rekindle relationships to get your life back on track.

Smiling directly influences other people's attitudes and how they respond to you. If you smile at a stranger, you will often receive a smile back. The more you smile the more positive reactions others will give you. Not just that, but it actually takes less physical energy to smile than frown.

Some people say that they have just forgotten how to smile. If you are one of these people, look at yourself in the mirror and give yourself a smile – you can't help but smile back.

REWRITING YOUR TRUTHS

Sometimes when we have felt the same way for a long time, the feeling becomes a belief for us, our truth if you like. We've all heard statements such as: *I always feel sore at night; I'll be like this forever; there's no relief in sight; my knee stops me from doing everything; I feel so old.* If you have been in a mindset that tells you that *you can't,* and then one day *you can,* you will need to re-write your truths: *I can do that; I had so much fun today that I didn't think about my pain as much; I can do much more than I ever thought I could.* This chapter explores the importance of acknowledging a change in your truths.

CHALLENGING YOUR TRUTHS

A statement, repeated often enough, becomes your truth. If it is negative, it becomes an unhelpful truth. Everything we know about living successfully with pain tells us that our thinking is vital to our success. So, as you use the strategies in this book and begin to find relief, you need to be aware of changing your truths to more helpful ones. Then, if you repeat them to yourself, over time, your new truths will become fact. A combination of positive thinking and pacing is the key.

This is a really powerful exercise, and one to which most people probably don't give much thought.

A teenage girl suffering from a painful debilitating

condition set a goal to attend her school camp. The camp was two weeks long and she wanted to attend for as much of that time as she could. While she tried to remain positive, she would occasionally have moments when she wondered if she could muster the stamina needed to be on camp. Before the camp, her truths sounded like this:

I always tire really easily,

I won't be able to keep up with the others and,

If I do too much, I will pay for it later with excruciating pain.

Despite these unhelpful truths, her determination to enjoy the school camp with her friends led her to pace herself and gradually increase her levels of activity to manageable amounts in preparation for the fortnight outdoors.

When the camp finally came around, the girl was able to participate in most of the activities and made sure she paced herself with enough rest breaks in between. At the end of the camp, she couldn't believe how much she had been able to do.

In a discussion with her teacher at the end of the camp, she reflected on how elated she was that she had done most of the things the other kids had done. Her teacher gently pointed out that her truths about herself now had to change because she had proven her existing truths wrong.

Wide-eyed, the girl suddenly understood. 'I can do these things,' she said in wonder. And with that statement, a world of possibilities opened up for her. If she *could* do the things that she thought she couldn't do, what other unhelpful truths could also be shattered? What if her truth became: *If I pace myself, I can do the same things the other kids do?* or *I had so much fun, I didn't even think about the pain.*

Think about the truths that you believe about yourself. Listen to yourself as you tell others your truths: *I can't walk up stairs because they'll cripple me* or *I can't sit for too long* or *I'll end up in hospital* or *I can't lift that, I'll end up in a wheelchair*. Listen to the truths of other people. Once you start listening, you'll hear people talk all the time about their limitations and the things that they've decided are true for them. Most of us fall so easily into creating unhelpful truths about ourselves that we forget about the more powerful helpful truths.

Like the girl on camp, experience can quickly change a truth. *I can't* becomes *I can*. If she had focused only on avoiding her pain, she never would have set the goal to go on camp. She had to give a little to get a lot. Her camp wasn't totally without pain, but she knew it was worth it to know that her dream of being with the other kids was possible.

Set some goals, start with manageable amounts, and use the strategies taught in this book to help you rewrite your truths.

PART 3

THE BEYOND PAIN PROGRAM

INTRODUCTION

This is it. The answer lies here. This program can help you change your life. The purpose of this program is to give you a choice: a choice to do what you want, when you want. A choice to say: *I could try that*, as opposed to: no *I can't do that*.

It focuses on what you *can do*, not what you can't. It focuses on what you want to achieve. It gives you tools and teaches you how to use them effectively to deal with your pain. It will make you your own pain management expert.

There is no pressure and no failure; this is just a program for you to follow, a program that allows the flexibility to do things at your own pace and not anyone else's.

This proven program will give you back control. It will empower you, and most importantly, it will teach you how to make decisions and tailor your rehabilitation to suit yourself.

Follow the program and you will reap the rewards.

I have used it.

My clients have used it.

It works.

JUST 8 WEEKS TO A NEW LIFE

Great things are not done by impulse, but by a series of small things brought together.

– Vincent Van Gogh

THIS PROGRAM WILL HELP YOU

People who follow this program have reported vast improvements in their quality of life. After just one week, all my clients begin to feel the benefit. After just four weeks, the change is remarkable. Incorporate these easy strategies into your daily life and you won't believe the difference. It really is possible.

> The first step is to *understand* your pain and *believe* in your ability.
> The second is to *set goals* so you know what to strive for.
> The third is to use these strategies to *manage* your pain and build your tolerances.

Like anything you do in the management of your health, if you are unsure, discuss this program with your doctor or treating health practitioner.

WHERE DO YOU START?

To make positive changes, a good place to start is to consider the things you *can* control. The past has passed. The future is unknown. The here-and-now is within your control. What are you going to do *today*?

Beyond Pain program

Step/Week	Strategy
1.	Acceptance and self-belief Pacing the day-to-day activities
2.	Setting goals Stretches
3.	Starting an exercise program and pacing up
4.	The right mindset
5.	Putting joy back into your life Keeping track
6.	Relaxation techniques
7.	A better night's sleep
8.	Managing flare-ups and setbacks

Take your time with these activities and understandings. There is no rush. Before you go on, ensure that you have read the second section of this book so that you will have a thorough understanding of your pain and the most effective strategies to deal with it. It will help you understand the program, the importance of having the right mindset and the benefits of gradually increasing your activity levels so that you are not pushing too hard or pushing through the pain.

If you find yourself in a lot of pain, stop. It is likely that you are pushing too hard, perhaps without even realising it. The key to all of the activities is that they should be *manageable* for you – even on a bad day. Of course, some strategies are going to be easier than others, and this will vary from person to person. But it is important to keep practising all of the strategies; do not limit yourself.

When things start to go well, try not to cut corners or become complacent. Don't try and do too much either. Stick to the program; it has been tested and proven to be effective, when done in its entirety.

You can ask your family and friends to support you. They may be able to help you stay motivated. A friend might go on walks with you. Your children or grandchildren might do some exercises with you. Doing exercises with other people will help you to stick to the program. Once you start the program and see the difference, you can change your life, and then maybe one day you will be in a position to change someone else's. You can help others improve their lives by sharing your positive experiences and showing them your improvement. If you have suffered for years and thought your situation could never change – and it does – then you will show everyone that anything is possible. This is an opportunity to inspire others through your own story.

This program will teach you how to get into the right mindset and how to set the numbers yourself. It's up to you how much or how little you do; you are in control. Don't compare yourself with others; everyone is different. Don't compare with your past; this is the here and now, and your circumstances have changed.

You can view instructional videos of the stretch and exercise programs, relaxation techniques, and download all of the worksheets for free by visiting www.beyondpain.com.au and navigating to the downloads page or by scanning the QR code.

WEEK 1

ACCEPTING AND BELIEVING

The first step towards managing your pain is accepting that you have pain and believing in your ability to take control of it. Yes, you have pain, *so now what are you going to do about it?*

Accepting your pain and believing in your ability is what will make the difference. Accepting your pain is not about giving up or losing hope – quite the contrary. Accepting your pain means you understand the following:

- that your journey might have been hard
- that you need to concentrate on the present using a positive mindset
- that it will take time and patience to bring about real change.

your pain is produced by your body

⇩

your body is controlled by your emotions and behaviour

⇩

your emotions and your behaviour are controlled by your thoughts

⇩

therefore, having helpful thoughts gives you the power to control your pain

⇩

this will allow your life to grow, leaving pain in your shadow

Not only do you need to accept your situation, but you also need to believe that you can change the way things are.

Self-belief is having confidence in your ability to take back control of your pain and your life. It is about believing that you will not let pain dictate what you do. It is about believing that real change is possible. The reality is that no matter how many strategies you learn, their effectiveness depends on your self-belief. It is not just about *doing* something; it is also about *believing* in what you are doing.

Accept your situation.

Believe that you can make your life better.

A lot of people ask what acceptance and self-belief might sound like. Here's what it sounds like in my pain clinic:

The more I do with my life, the less I notice my pain.

I'm in the driver's seat, not the pain.

I've got this pain, but I'm going to live my normal life anyway.

I may have flare-ups, but I know it will be temporary and I will deal with it.

The pain is not me. It's a small part of me that I deal with.

Acceptance and self-belief are the foundations for a purposeful life of happiness and achievement. When you have these foundations, things *will* change.

AFFIRMATIONS

Affirmations are positive statements that help motivate you. They are a great start to help you accept your situation and believe in your own abilities. Many people use affirmations to great effect. They work best when they are repeated regularly while looking into a mirror. They should always be phrased in a positive way. Here are some that you might use:

- *I will be able to do all of my exercises today.*
- *I will take my time and finish the shopping.*
- *I can weed half the garden.*
- *I will be able to walk all the way to the shops by the end of the week.*
- *Every day I take more control.*

Affirmations

- Choose two affirmations or think of your own.
- Write them on a post-it note on your mirror or at work on your desk.
- Repeat these affirmations regularly to help you believe in a better future.
- Build affirmations into your daily routine.
- Say them at least twice a day. Looking in the mirror while you say them is best.

At first, they might sound like a lie, but when you embrace this method, one morning you will say them, and you will truly believe them. This technique is tried and tested and it really works. The key is to have patience and persevere.

Be wary of unhelpful affirmations such as:

- *I will get rid of my pain.*
- *There is a cure out there; I just need to find it.*
- *I have to push through this pain.*

Philosopher Elbert Hubbert once said: 'A failure is a man who has blundered but is unable to cash in on the experience.' It is up to you to cash in on your experience, accept your situation and believe in your ability to have a brighter future.

PACING UP DAY-TO-DAY ACTIVITIES (ACTIVITY-RELAX CYCLE)

There is no benefit in overdoing things; gradually pacing up is the best option. Do this by starting with *manageable* amounts of activity that you can do *comfortably* and *confidently*, and then gradually increasing (pace up) the amounts.

A manageable amount is an amount where you may feel slightly more pain, or a different sensation altogether, but it doesn't have to be. If you're a numbers person, a manageable amount is about 65-75% of your current maximum tolerance. Essentially, it is an amount that you feel comfortable or confident with; an amount where there is still a buffer or reserve of energy.

Just say you want to clean your house. You might find thirty minutes of housework very painful, but confident with doing twenty minutes. So, twenty minutes will be your manageable amount. After twenty minutes, stop cleaning and do something else, something less active and more relaxing. You might have a cup of tea, watch TV, or read a magazine for ten minutes before getting back to another twenty minutes of cleaning. This is called an activity-relax cycle. Over time, you gradually pace up your activity amount.

Your activity-relax cycle needs to have a combination of both activity *and* relaxation. However, the relaxation period does not mean that you have to be completely inactive; it can be something *less* active. For example, if your activity was jogging, then your relaxation period might be walking at a gentle pace, or stopping to do a few quick stretches.

A good way of understanding what works best for you is to make a note of your activity-relax cycle and monitor your progress. Making notes about your progress will allow you to recognise and celebrate your achievements. For example, in the first week you might have cleaned for twenty minutes then relaxed for ten minutes. Two weeks later, you might be able to clean for twenty-five minutes and only need to relax for five.

THINGS TO CONSIDER

Don't do something active like cleaning the house and then decide that your relaxation period should be pushing a wheelbarrow in the garden. Both of these require you to be physically active. The reverse is also true. If your activity is sitting and working on the computer, then your relaxation period shouldn't be sitting on the couch and watching TV, rather completing a few stretches or getting up and going for a walk.

It is all about pacing and increasing your activity amounts gradually either weekly or fortnightly, irrespective of your pain levels. A good amount is about a 20-25% increase on your activity amount. And remember, some of this will be trial and error. Sometimes you will need to test the waters to fully understand how this works. Be a little conservative when you try things. Sometimes when you are active, your feel-good hormones act on the pain traffic lights and masks the pain. If you begin gently, any increases in pain will be kept to a minimum. In other words, don't do what I did when I climbed the 1,000 steps of Mt Dandenong. After my over-enthusiasm, I suffered for a week.

Stick to the plan and only pace up your activity amounts on a weekly basis. Even if you feel good, relax when it's time to, and give your body that extra bit of breathing space to enjoy doing the activity without feeling the struggle afterwards. Don't fall into the trap of doing more and pushing to your limits if it feels good.

It's a bit like driving a car. If you refuel every time the fuel gauge goes to quarter full, you will never get stranded. But if you keep pushing it until the low-fuel light comes on, you will one day get stranded.

Remember that using the activity-relax cycle will allow you to achieve your goals in a more enjoyable and rewarding way. In turn, it will also give you the confidence that you can do it.

HEAT & ICE PACKS

Just like pacing activities, the notion of little-and-often also applies here. Many clients say they use heat and/or ice to help manage symptoms, but most either sit with an ice pack on at the end of the day or go to bed with a heat pack.

What would be more useful is to use heat or ice five or six times per day, but only for up to five minutes at a time, even when you feel good: little-and-often. For example, have it on when you eat your meals, watch TV, and, before or after some exercise. Doing it in short bursts means it won't interrupt your daily routine, and it will help reduce the build-up of your symptoms through the day.

A common question people ask is which is better: heat or ice? This is a tough question to answer because it depends on the person and the circumstances but generally speaking, if your painful part feels stiff and sore, then heat is likely to help; if it feels hot and swollen, then use ice. A bit of trial-and-error will be needed here. Of course, make sure the pack is either warm or cool, not hot or cold. This way you're less likely to get burnt!

REMINDERS

To stop you from doing too much or too little, it is helpful to have reminders to monitor your manageable amounts. Internal reminders come from your body and they help you to be more aware of your body. Is your soreness worsening? Are you becoming stiffer? Are you starting to get frustrated? Being more aware, allows you to implement your activity-relax cycles more effectively.

Your external reminders are like a timer on your mobile phone or on your computer, or something that you can see or hear that will remind you to change position. Pacing to a manageable amount is a skill you need to learn. Using the reminders will help make it a habit.

Some examples:

Work	If you work in an office, you might find that sitting for 30 minutes causes you a lot of pain, but 20 minutes is a comfortable amount. So for your activity-relax cycle, you could do your work for 20 minutes and then get up and do a few stretches or go for a quick walk before sitting down again. You can use your mobile phone or an alarm on your computer to remind you to pace yourself. Each week, you can pace up the amount of time you spend sitting, say by 10 minutes, to gradually build up your tolerances.
Gardening	You may find that you have a lot of pain after an hour of heavy gardening. For your activity-rest cycle, you may decide to do 40 minutes of gardening and then do a few easy trimmings or just relax with a drink for 20 minutes before you get back to it. You may use a timer to keep track. Every week, you can pace up the amount of gardening by five minutes to improve your tolerances.

Cinemas	A manageable amount of sitting for you may be 20 minutes. So, to implement an activity-relax cycle, find a seat near an aisle and put your mobile phone alarm on vibrate for every 20 minutes to remind you to stand, stretch and then sit back down.
Housework	You may be able to vacuum one room comfortably. To implement an activity-relax cycle, you could vacuum one room then do some light dusting or just take a break for five minutes before starting vacuuming the next room. Each week, you can pace up the length of time you spend vacuuming.
Cooking	Your manageable amount of standing while cooking may be 30 minutes. So for your activity-relax cycle, you might decide to cut the vegies while standing, then sit on a stool for five minutes while you stir the vegies on the stove, and then stand again for the next part. You may use a small oven timer as reminder.
Driving	Your driving tolerance may be 30 minutes before you are in a lot of pain. But you may be able to drive comfortably for 20 minutes. To successfully implement an activity-relax cycle, you can drive for 20 minutes, then pull over, get out, walk around the car, do a few stretches and then get back on the road again. It may take you a bit longer to reach your destination, but you won't be in agony when you get there.

THE WEEKLY PLANNER

Many clients find it very useful to plan and then track their progress. So, I recommend you do a weekly planner. A weekly planner is useful because it gives you an idea of what to expect in the week ahead, allows you to change anything if need be, and then monitor it as the days go by. Essentially, it allows you to be proactive rather than reactive.

Over the weekend, write down what you have planned for each day of the upcoming week. Things like when you plan to get up, have your meals, your appointments, daily chores, exercises, enjoyable activities and so on. Anything that you have planned for the week should be written in your planner. It should not take more than one hour to complete; that's one hour, once per week. If you already use a planner, great.

As each day goes by, I recommend you tick off activities you have completed and cross off those you didn't. Write brief notes where unexpected things came up, when your pain changed after completing something, or why you didn't get around to doing something. It may also help to write how you felt overall for the day. Remember, don't just write about when things are worse; also write about when things are better.

This way, you will be able to see what went well and what didn't, and, most importantly, identify any patterns in your symptoms.

One client completed a weekly planner for three weeks. When she first came into the clinic, she declared: 'I feel most pain when I'm trying to relax!' When she completed her planner, we noticed that she was working a shift as a carer for the elderly, then going home to rest as her pain increased. This allowed her to see the link between her work patterns and a delayed pain response. So, to be proactive, in the subsequent planners, we planned and implemented some relaxation strategies during her shift. Not surprisingly, she reported less pain.

The planner also gave her confidence because it allowed her to review the other days in advance and make suitable adjustments; she knew exactly what she was going to be doing.

A weekly planner may look like this:

Weekly Planner (Please include approximate time you will do activity ; eg. *shopping 1pm-2pm*)

	Monday	Tuesday	Wednesday	Thursday	Friday	Saturday	Sunday
Morning (5am – 12pm)	Get up 8am	Get up 8am	Get up 8am	Get up 8am	Get up 8am	Get up 9am	Get up 9am
	Drop kids	Drop kids 8:30am	Drop kids at 8.30	Drop kids	Drop kids	BREAKFAST	BREAKFAST
	BREAKFAST	BREAKFAST	BREAKFAST	BREAKFAST	BREAKFAST	Spend time with Kids	Walk
	Walk	Brief walk / lie down	Read books	Gardening	Go to Bank / Shopping	rest	rest
	Rest		Walk\ lie down	rest			
Afternoon (12pm-5pm)	LUNCH	LUNCH	LUNCH	LUNCH	LUNCH	LUNCH	LUNCH
	Read books	Exercises	GP appointment	Shopping	Pick up kids	Gardening	Exercise
	Pick up kids	Enjoyable activity	Hydrotherapy	Pick up kids	Read books	Enjoy some time relaxing	Go out with kids and family
	Exercise	Meditation/ Mindfulness	Pick up kids	Computer work	Pick up kids		
	Rest	Pick up kids			Rest	Grocery shopping	
Evening (5pm-10pm)	Drop kids at sport	Drop kids at music	Drop kids at sport	Walk	Go out to drinks and DINNER	Computer work	Read books
	DINNER	Hydrotherapy	DINNER	DINNER	Check emails	DINNER	Walk
	Watch TV	DINNER	Meditation	Meditation/ Mindfulness	Meditation	Meditation/ Mindfulness	DINNER
	Bed	Bed	Bed	Bed	Bed	Bed	Relax
							Bed

Sometimes you may be concerned that you won't be able to stick to your plan. That's okay, accept that unexpected things do happen and just stick to the plan to the best of your ability. The thing is that a weekly planner, aside from allowing you to be proactive, will also allow you see your own progress towards taking control of your life and achieving your goals. It will also help you to rejoice in your gains. You might look back over your first couple of weeks and read that you found shopping difficult, and realise that now, you don't.

- Write two affirmations on post-it notes and place them where you can use them as reminders.
- Think about the different activities in your life now: work, cleaning, cooking, gardening and so on. Think of how you can incorporate an activity-relax cycle into these activities. Use the activity-relax cycle for at least three activities.
- Remember, don't overdo it. Pick an amount of activity that is *manageable* to start with – an amount with which you are comfortable and confident.
- Do a weekly planner for the week ahead.
- Remember to also record your activity-relax cycles.

BY THE END OF THE FIRST WEEK...

You might notice patterns that show progress. You might have considered more activities for the second week. If you normally tend to overdo things, you might have considered less activities for the second week. You might have also noticed a change in the way that you are listing your feelings. You might have felt better or more confident by the end of the first week. You may have begun to understand how you can still have the pain, and do more. You might not have noticed your pain quite as much. You might have had no increase in pain despite the changes in your activity levels, and the activity-relax cycles may have become easier to do as the week progressed. The key to a successful first week is to get into the right mindset and understand the concept of *manageable* amounts of activity.

WEEK 2

GOAL SETTING

For all sufferers of chronic pain..... To identify some useful goals, it is helpful to have a brainstorming session, and separate the goals into three columns: personal, social, and vocational/volunteer. To me, these columns represent the three pillars of life. They work as a triad; a *life triad*. So, if you have a goal to lose weight, put this in the personal column; if your goal is to have dinner with friends, put this in the social column; and if you wanted to do some part-time or volunteer work at some stage, put this in the vocational/volunteer column.

Brainstorming

Imagine you don't have any pain.

- What would you like to do?
- Think of activities you have enjoyed in the past that you would like to do again.
- Think of activities that you would like to start, including those you never imagined you could do.
- Activities can range from playing contact sports, to reading a book to going dancing
- Write down a list and pick four goals to work on: two you need to do, and two you would enjoy doing. Remember, the focus is on improving your activity so make sure some of your goals also involve physical activity.
- Don't hold back on your ideas. Think of what you would really like to do if you didn't have the pain at all.

Look at your list. The best goals need to be specific, measurable and achievable. But, as a start, take a few of things you want to work on from the brainstorming session. For example, they may be:

- to play a game of golf
- to take my grandchildren to the zoo
- to go ballroom dancing with my partner.

For those of you who have never set goals before, in order to have a clear sense of direction, a really easy way is to use the SMART method.

SMART GOALS

SMART Goals

S = specific
M = measurable
A = achievable
R = relevant or meaningful
T = timed

A SMART goal might look something like this:

- To play nine holes of golf by 12th April.

It is *specific* because it is nine holes of golf.
It is *measurable* because you specified how many holes you want to play.
It is *achievable* because you intend to take the necessary steps to achieve it.
It is *relevant* and *meaningful* because you love golf and the outdoors.
You have *timed* the task to ensure you achieve the goal by 12th April.

All goals need to have the five SMART goal elements. Sometimes this is easy, and sometimes it can present difficulties to people with chronic pain. You can also incorporate the following strategies to help.

Worksheets can be found at the back of this book, by scanning the QR code, or by visiting www.beyondpain.com.au and navigating to the 'Downloads' page.

MOUNTAINS AND CHECK-POINTS

I climbed a literal mountain when I went to the base camp of Everest, but I couldn't have achieved that goal without breaking it down into shorter chunks. You don't have to climb a real mountain to find the metaphor useful.

- Think of your long-term goal as the mountain
- Break down the goal into shorter chunks. These are the check-points along the way

Long-term goal *The mountain*	Short-term goals *The check-points*
To attend a short course on computers for two days a week (1ˢᵗ May)	1. Increase sitting tolerance up to 45 minutes to manage public transport, lectures and classes (by 10th April). 2. Improve concentration by reading daily (by 17th April). 3. Improve standing tolerance to 30 minutes (by 10th April). 4. Improve carrying a backpack (<5 kg) for one hour (by 17th April). 5. Discuss availability of seating with the course organisers (by 3rd April).

Long-term goal *The mountain*	Short-term goals *The check-points*
Be able to cook Christmas dinner for the extended family (in six weeks' time)	1. Build up the strength in the hand and arm muscles to cook a range of simple meals (by 26th November). 2. Improve standing and reaching times and bending to put things in the oven (by 8th December). 3. Practice different types of grip for chopping and peeling and holding trays (8th December). 4. Practice roasting smaller items that are lighter to carry (15th December). 5. Continue stretching and exercise program (as per plan).
Play nine holes of golf (25th June)	1. Go to the driving range twice a week to practice swinging a golf club (by 30th May). 2. Practice putting every Saturday morning. 3. Walk daily and building up my walking tolerance to be able to walk for one hour (by 9th May) 4. Play golf for two hours (by 16th May) 5. Continue to do my exercises to build the strength in my back (as per exercise plan).

You might find it easier to achieve your goals if you involve others. With the example involving golf, set the date for a game with friends, or talk with others about what you are planning.

If you are looking at a particular goal and your first thought started with *I could never do that,* here is a strategy that could help, particularly if the goal causes you anxiety or worry at the thought of trying to achieve it. It involves breaking the goal down into achievable smaller components. Remember, a house is built brick by brick.

The 10-step goal sheet

- List your goal at number 10 and list nine smaller steps, each one a little more challenging than the previous.
- Each step has a 0 to100% confidence rating (where 0% is no confidence and 100% is complete confidence). The idea is that you repeat step 1 until your confidence level rises above 70% while you perform the step before you progress to step 2. It is normal to have some anxiety in the achievement steps towards your goal. I recommend 70% because I recognise this and it means that you are experiencing more feelings of confidence than anxiety. In other words, you've tipped the scales.
- You then stay on step 2 until your confidence is more than 70% then progress to step 3. Let your confidence levels dictate when you move on to the next step.
- This continues until you reach step 10 – your goal.

For example, say your goal is to Return to work part time, working three full days as a truck driver. Your 10-step goal sheet may look something like this:

Step	Steps to achieving the goal	Confidence rating (0–100%)
1	Increase your sitting tolerance in a car to 30 minutes	
2	Increase your sitting tolerance in a car to 1 hour of driving	
3	Increase your sitting tolerance in a car to 2 hours of driving	
4	Speak with your employer regarding suitable work options	
5	Be a passenger in a truck for two half days per week	
6	Be a passenger three half days per week	
7	Be a passenger on a part-time basis, three full days per week	

Step	Steps to achieving the goal	Confidence rating (0–100%)
8	Drive a truck two half days per week	
9	Drive a truck two full days	
10	Returning to work part-time, working three full days as a truck driver	

Note: It is okay for the order to change or extra steps to be added. The 10-step plan is a guide, and once you start, you may realise that you need to modify the plan slightly. Everyone is different.

STAYING FOCUSED

While coming up with a goal can be difficult, staying focused on achieving the goal often poses a greater challenge. Many of my clients have mentioned this to me, but I didn't truly understand until I experienced it myself. Following my burns, setting the goal of returning to work wasn't difficult because I really wanted my life back, but staying focused was a different story. There were times when it all felt too hard, and it would have been easier to give up. I started to make excuses and procrastinate – *I will just watch this movie and get back to it*, or *I will start tomorrow*.

To help you stay focused, try the following:

- Set a clear plan in your logbook outlining how you will achieve the goal, and review this plan on a weekly basis, so that you know exactly what needs to be done to move forward. Your plan needs to include details of when you will work on your goal and for how long, as well as listing your long-term and short-term goals.

- Tell other people about your goal so that they can encourage you through the process, and so that you feel a sense of honouring your word.
- When things seem *too* difficult, or you experience a flare-up, remind yourself of why you have set the goal, how far you have come, and what it means to achieve your goal. To help, close your eyes and imagine how it would feel, both physically and emotionally, to achieve your goal. You can also try listening to inspiring music or watch an inspirational movie or documentary.
- Track your progress in your logbook by making a note every time you make a gain towards your goal, no matter how small.
- You may want to make a series of short videos as you work towards your goal. You can then upload these videos on websites such as YouTube (www.youtube.com) or GiveIt100 (www.giveit100.com) to document your progress and share your achievements with friends and family. In my clinic, I video my clients doing activities such as walking and lifting, before and after they complete the Beyond Pain program, to help them reflect on their achievements. And if they are happy for me to do so, I upload a short video to the internet and provide them with a link.

CELEBRATE

As important as it is to set goals and work towards them, it is just as important that you recognise and acknowledge what you have achieved. Take the time to recognise your achievement. Make a point to celebrate it. When you do this, the first thing you think about is setting a new goal while patting yourself on the back for doing something you didn't think you could.

For people with chronic pain, sometimes the goals might not seem like much – being able to hold the kettle to make a cup of tea, sit in the car long enough to drive to the local shops, wearing high heels to a party – but they are huge. Never forget to pat yourself on the back. See each small step as a part of a much larger journey, a small piece of a much bigger picture, a small step for most, a giant leap for you.

STRENGTHENING YOUR AFFIRMATIONS

To further help you believe in your ability to achieve your goals, you can build on your affirmations to be more effective. Try extending them to be more powerful by turning them into a question that you have to answer. Instead of the affirmation: *I will be able to manage my work*, change it to: *Why will I be able to manage my work?*

It might seem like a small difference, but the question asks you to list achievements in response. Your answer to the question *Why will I be able to manage my work?* might sound something like this: *I can manage my work because I am learning new ways by reading this book. I am building up my tolerance to sitting at my desk. I have kept up with my exercises and feel fitter. I can use relaxation techniques. I feel like I'm taking back control of my life.*

One woman at my clinic was very excited by her progress after the first three weeks.

'I'm doing so well and I feel so wonderful that I don't want to progress my exercises just in case I go backwards,' she declared after one visit.

Because her improvements were entirely due to following the gentle exercise program and changing her beliefs about herself and what she could do, I used affirmation questioning to help her to challenge this new belief before it became ingrained.

'Why will you continue to improve if you progress your

exercises further?' I asked her. To my relief, she switched her thinking immediately.

'Well I guess that it's the exercises that have gotten me to this point, so maybe if I continued them, my body would get stronger and then I would be more flexible and I would be able to do more things.'

'Exactly,' I said, grinning. She got it.

Affirming questions

- Think of the affirmations you've been using, or think of a couple of new ones.
- Change the affirmations into questions, and record them in your logbook.

Affirmation	Affirming question
I will be able to play a game of golf	Why will I be able to play a game of golf?
I am in the driver's seat	Why am I in the driver's seat?
I can take control of my pain	Why can I take control of my pain?

- Place it with your affirmations on the post-it notes or replace your affirmation with the questions. Ask yourself the questions daily.
- Record in your logbook how you felt before and after you have done them.

Initially, you may not have the answers to your affirmation questions, and this is okay. Simply pose the questions and the answers will come as you follow this program.

STRETCHING

Stretching is a vital component in pain management. Stretching improves the health of your tissues, muscles, bones and even your nerves. When you stretch, it is important that you do it gently, smoothly and in a relaxed manner. Don't push or force yourself.

Three typical signs that you are pushing or forcing a stretch are:
- holding your breath and then grunting or groaning
- clenching your fists or shrugging your shoulders
- gritting your teeth in effort or your body shaking

If you notice yourself doing any of these then you need to stop, relax for a moment and then focus on staying relaxed as you do the stretch again. Too much muscle tension will only worsen your pain.

Stretching

Stretches need to be done in a gentle, smooth and a relaxed manner. Remember what is manageable for you.
- Do your stretch program once a day (any time of day is fine).
- Warm up first, following the warm-up guide below.
- Do each stretch to a count of 5 to start with.
- Increase by one count daily until you reach a count of 10.
- Once you have reached a count of 10, keep it at that.

The key to effective stretches is to not stretch beyond your manageable limits. Stretches should be in a good challenging range; they shouldn't cause unmanageable pain. You'll know when you reach your manageable limits because you will feel a greater stretch and a slight increase in pain (maybe even a slight tingling or a pins-and-needles sensation).

The key here is that you shouldn't push yourself; do only what is manageable. If a stretch seems too difficult now, leave it for now and come back to it in a week or two.

WARMING UP

Before you stretch, you must warm up properly. This will make the stretches more effective and prepare your body so that you are less likely to injure yourself.

Warm-ups are done while standing, with feet shoulder width apart.

WARM-UP		FREQUENCY
The Nod	Gently look up and then down.	5 times
The Spectator	Turn your head gently from side to side, like a spectator watching a rally in tennis.	5 times
The Nodding Spectator	While looking up and down, gently turn your head from side to side. It's like watching a bouncing kangaroo go past very slowly. Your head nods gently up and down while you slowly turn your head from left to right, and then right to left. Another way to describe it is to imagine you are watching someone on a pogo stick going past in slow motion.	5 times

WARM-UP		FREQUENCY
The Shoulder Circles	Circle or rotate your shoulders forward and then back.	5 each direction
Leg Slaps	Let your arms hang loose by your side. While twisting your back, let your arms swing around and flop against your thighs or buttocks as you twist.	5 each direction
Upper Back Rotations	Lift your elbows out to your sides as far as you can manage and twist your body from side to side to loosen your upper back.	5 each direction

STRETCHES

Do each stretch for a count of 5. Increase by one count every day until you reach a count of 10. When you reach a count of 10, focus on increasing the range of movement within each stretch.

Remember, stretches should be done to your manageable level. If you find yourself holding your breath, gritting your teeth or tensing up your muscles, adjust the stretch so that you're comfortable again. If you still find it too difficult, leave it and come back to it in a week or two.

The stretches are done in three positions: sitting, lying and standing. If you find a position difficult, just take your time and do what you can for each stretch. It's important to make a start somewhere. Doing a little bit of each is better than not doing them at all. Just remember the stretching motto: gently, smoothly and in a relaxed manner.

SITTING STRETCHES

Sit down on a firm chair with a back rest but no arm supports. Ensure that you can place your feet comfortably on the floor

	1. Spread your fingers apart. Hold the stretch for the count.
	2. Place both of your palms together as if you are praying. Keeping your palms together, lift your elbows up towards the level of your shoulders. Hold the stretch for the count.
	3. Place the backs of your hands together with your fingers pointing down. Keeping the backs of your hands together, lower your elbows towards your waist. Hold the stretch for the count.
	4. Use your right hand and gently pull the fingers of your left hand back. Hold each stretch for the count and then do the same on the other side.

	5. Take your left arm across your body towards your right shoulder. Use your right hand and push your left elbow further towards the right shoulder. Hold for the count and then repeat on the other side.
	6. Place both of your hands on the back of your head. Keeping your elbows pointing forward, tuck your chin in and lean back against the back rest. Hold for the count.
	7. Place both of your hands on the back of your head. Keeping your elbows pointing forward, curl yourself so that you bring your head and elbows towards your waist. Keep your back rested against the back of the chair. Hold for the count.
	8. Hold the right side of the chair with your right hand. Lean to the left and use your left hand to guide your head further to the left. You will feel a stretch on the right side of your neck. Hold for the count and then repeat on the other side.
	9. Hold the right side of the chair with your right hand. Turn your head to the left. Lean to the left and use your left hand to guide the head further towards your left underarm. You will feel a stretch down the back of your neck. Hold for the count and then repeat on the other side.

	10. Lean back on the chair. Let your arms dangle behind you and bring your chest forward. Look upwards to stretch the front of your body. You can rotate your hands outwards so your palms are facing up for a greater stretch. Hold for the count.
	11. Take your right hand and place it on your left knee. Turn your body to the left and use your left hand to touch the back of the chair. Hold for the count and then repeat on the other side.

LYING STRETCHES

Lie down on your back on a flat surface. You can use a mat or firm mattress for comfort. If you find it difficult to lie on your back, take a short break between the stretches.

	1. Point your toes and reach your arms over your head to make yourself as long as possible. Hold for the count
	2. Bend both knees up towards your chest. Use your hands to help you. Hold for the count
	3. Bend your knees and rest your feet on the floor. Cross your right leg over your left and ensure that there are no gaps between your thighs. Bring both knees up towards your chest. Use your arms to help you. Hold for the count and then repeat with your left leg over your right leg.

	4. Bend your knees with your feet together on the floor. While keeping your knees together, wriggle your feet apart. Let your knees fall inwards and feel the stretch deep in your hips. Hold the stretch for the count.
	5. Bend your knees with your feet on the floor. Keeping your knees and feet together, place your arms out to the sides like the wings of an aeroplane. Roll both knees to one side and then to the other side. You don't need to hold this stretch, but repeat each side to the count. For example, roll your knees to each side five times.
	6. Sit on the floor with your legs straight. Bend your right knee up and cross it over your left leg. Place your left elbow or forearm on your right knee and turn to the right and place your right hand behind you by turning to the side of the bent knee. Hold the stretch for the count and then repeat on the other side.
	7. While sitting up straight, bring both of your feet together towards you. Hold onto your ankles and drop your knees outwards. You can use your forearms and elbows to push your knees apart until you feel the stretch. Hold for the count.
	8. Lie on your front with your arms out straight. Push down with your palms and look up by lifting your head and neck. Don't hold this stretch, but repeat lifting your head up and then down for the count.

	9. Lie on your front. Bend one knee up and use your hands to hold your ankle or the end of your trousers. Hold for the count and repeat on the other side. If you can't reach, just bend your knee as far as you can manage.
	10. Get onto your hands and knees and ensure that you are not resting on your toes. Gently walk your hands back so that you are sitting on your heels. Walk your hands further behind you and lift your pelvis forward. Hold for the count. If you cannot walk your hands back, simply try to sit on your heels.
	11. Get onto your hands and knees. Keeping your arms out straight, sit back on your heels and lower your head. Hold for the count..

STANDING STRETCHES

Stand with your feet apart and your toes pointing forward.

	1. Start with your hands by your side, palms facing inwards. Bring your arms out to the side to shoulder level. If you can't get them this high, that can be a goal as you improve. Hold for the count.

	2. Start with hands by your side, you're your arms rotated outwards so your palms are facing out. Bring your arms out to the side to shoulder level with your palms facing up. Then tilt your hands downwards, so that your fingertips are pointing towards the floor. Hold for the count.
	2. Start with hands by your side, your arms rotated outwards so your palms are facing out.
	4. Move your right arm down the side of your right leg, bending your upper body to the right. Bring your left arm up and over. Hold for the count and then repeat on the other side.
	5. Keep both feet pointing forward. Take a step forward with your right leg. Keeping your left knee straight, bend your right knee. Hold for the count and then repeat on the other side.

	6. Keep both feet pointing forward. Take a large step forward with your right foot. Keep your left knee straight and turn your left foot outwards (quarter turn). Bend your front knee and stretch the inner part of your back leg. Hold for the count and then repeat on the other side.
	7. Slowly bend forward towards your feet in a relaxed manner and then back up again. Don't hold this stretch, but repeat down and then up for the count. For example, go down and then up five times.
	8. Place your hands on your buttocks. Keep your legs straight and push your waist forward. Don't hold this stretch, but repeat forward and back for the count. For example, push back and then forward five times.
	9. Place your hands on the upper part of your back. Roll your shoulders back, and roll your shoulders forward. Repeat the rolling forward and back motion for the count. For example, roll forward and back five times.

Take your time getting used to the stretches. When you are more confident, you will do them a lot faster. They will only take about 20 minutes, but in the first week, while you're getting used to them, they will take a bit longer.

Everyone is different, but most people feel more supple after doing these stretches for a week. If the stretching exercises cause an increase in your pain, do them slower or don't stretch as far. Remember, if you have been inactive for a while, physical activity may cause some muscle soreness. This is completely normal for anyone, not just people with chronic pain.

The stretch program video can be viewed for free by scanning the QR code, or by visiting www.beyondpain.com.au and navigating to the 'Downloads' page.

Weekly review

- Commence the stretch program remembering your manageable limits and that the stretches are to be done gently, smoothly and in a relaxed manner.
- Keep a daily record in your logbook of what you do, how you feel and what you think.
- Write affirmation questions on post-it notes and place them where you can use them as reminders. Record them in your logbook. Continue using your affirmations.
- Complete a brainstorming session for your goals and list four long-term goals. Ensure that they are a combination of things you enjoy and things you feel you need to do. Ensure that they follow the SMART principle: specific, measurable, achievable, relevant, and timed.
- For each goal, break it into a series of short-term goals or fill out a 10-step goal sheet so that you have a plan. Make a start on the ones you can.

And continue...

- Thinking about how you can increase your activity amounts for the second week and whether there are any daily activities you can incorporate into the activity-relax cycle.
- Being aware of your body and focus on the gains, no matter how little.
- Pacing to an amount or time, not pain.

WEEK 3

GETTING STARTED ON EXERCISE

To begin your exercises, you need to first establish a starting point for each exercise. A starting point is a manageable amount: an amount with which you are comfortable and confident with.

Your starting point is typically an amount that you can do:

- without pushing through too much pain
- without added tension
- without stopping too soon
- where you may feel a different pain or sensation.

Try each exercise and for each, identify an amount that is manageable for you. Record these in your exercise chart (the template can be found at the back of this book or downloaded for free by going to www.beyondpain.com.au and clicking on the 'Products & Downloads' tab).

These amounts will be your starting point. Your exercises need to be done three times a week. To do this, follow these simple steps:

1. Choose three days that suit you. This will allow you to allocate enough time for your exercises by giving you a snapshot of when you need to do them.
2. Write the starting points for the exercises under each of the three days. You will be keeping these numbers the same for the whole week. See the example below. Think of it like a worker filling out their shifts on the roster for the upcoming week.

	Week 1 of exercise				
	Mon	Tues	Wed	Thurs	Fri
Arm Circles (max 2 mins)	20 secs	Break	20 secs	Break	20 secs
Side Leans (max 10)	3	Break	3	Break	3
Lunge Squats (max 15)	2	Break	2	Break	2

3. Once you have filled out the numbers for all the exercises, have a look at your chart. If you are not happy with the numbers because you think it looks unmanageable, change them. But once you are satisfied with what you have written, stick to the plan; don't change it mid-week. Remember, it is always better to be conservative and build up than going hard and crashing.

4. Find time to do all of your exercises in one go so that you will not only increase your strength, but also your endurance.

5. As you complete the exercises on each day, put a tick next to them. The tick is important because it is a visual reward to recognise your achievement. See the example below.

	Week 1 of exercise				
	Mon	Tues	Wed	Thurs	Fri
Arm Circles (max 2 mins)	20 secs ✓	Break	20 secs ✓	Break	20 secs ✓
Side Leans (max 10)	3 ✓	Break	3 ✓	Break	3 ✓
Lunge Squats (max 15)	2 ✓	Break	2 ✓	Break	2 ✓

Your exercise record might look like the grid above at the end of the first week. The numbers on this plan are just examples, not recommendations. You need to try the exercises, determine your comfort levels and set your own numbers. Everyone is different. Everyone's pain levels are different. Only you will know what you can do comfortably.

By doing the exercises you will know what your manageable amounts are. Complete the first week, and then reflect on how you went in order to decide what to do in the second week.

At the end of the first week, especially if you haven't exercised for a long time, you might feel some increase in your pain levels. This is completely normal. The discomfort you feel is called *training pain*. It is your body's way of saying that it is not used to what it is being put through. Some people even refer to it as *good pain*. This pain is not a sign of damage or harm, and it cannot be avoided, but it will reduce gradually as you exercise regularly. As you get more confident with your exercises you will learn to do them faster and gain great health benefits, not just strength.

Remember, not everyone will feel this training pain because everyone is different. But if you do feel an increase in pain, you be the judge. If it is a slight increase from your normal pain level, it's nothing to worry about. If it is more than a slight increase, then your starting points might be too high. Pain is not a sign to avoid exercise; you just need to figure out suitable start points. You can also progress very slowly the following week.

If you are worried about wear and tear, don't be. Our joints, muscles, tendons and ligaments need movement to stay healthy. A lack of movement can result in just as much wear and tear as overdoing it can; remember that lubrication of the joints occurs when we move them.

In the weeks ahead, keep in mind that the best benefits occur when you regularly and gradually increase the amounts you do.

EXERCISES

Now for the exercises. Try each one to establish your start points. You will find some easier than others depending on where your pain is.

Some of the exercises require you to repeat on the left and the right side. Lunges are an example of this. If you can do four on one side, but six on the other side, use the lower amount as your start-point for the first week.

When you complete all of the exercises, your whole body will benefit. They are designed to work all your muscle groups. Remember, even if they are awkward and difficult to begin with, you will soon be doing them with ease.

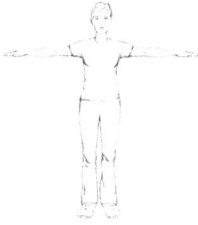

Arm circles

Stand with your feet apart. Raise your arms to the side as far as you can manage, no higher than shoulder level. Keeping your arms straight, make small gentle circles forwards and record the time or count the number of circles. Then make small gentle circles backwards for the same time or count. Be conservative to start with.

Maximum time 2 minutes or 40 circles: you can progress by holding weights.

This exercise builds the endurance in your shoulders and upper back.

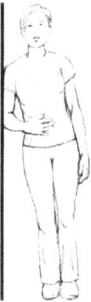

Side leans

Stand sideways next to a wall. Make sure your feet are about 20 cm away from the wall so that you are leaning slightly. Rest your shoulder against the wall and rest your hand closest to the wall on your stomach. Keep your shoulder against the wall and move your hip towards the wall in a gentle motion and then back out again. You don't need to touch the wall with your hip.

Maximum 10: you can progress by moving your feet further away from the wall.

This exercise is helpful in strengthening your hips and increasing their flexibility.

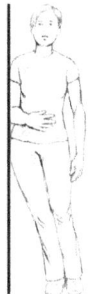

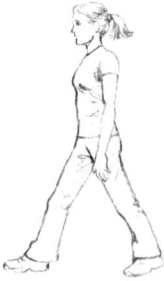

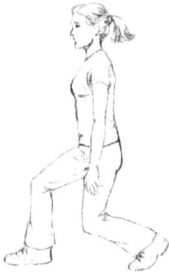

Lunge squat

Stand with your feet shoulder width apart. Take a step forward with one leg (as far as you can manage). Ensure that both of your feet are pointing forward. Bend both knees and lower your waist and your back knee straight down. Try to keep your front knee still (often it will move forward). Return to the standing position then take another step with the same leg and repeat the lunge squat. Once you have completed one side, repeat on the other side.

Maximum 15: you can progress by holding onto weights.

This exercise is great for core stability, balance and strengthening your legs and buttocks.

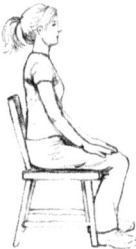

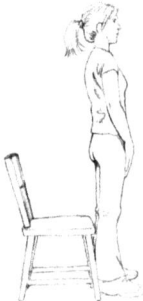

Sit to stands

Sit with your legs a little apart on a firm chair with a back support. Keeping your feet flat on the floor, tighten your buttocks and stand up using your leg muscles. Try to not use your hands to push off.

Sometimes your knees come together when you sit or stand. Try to prevent your knees from coming together by concentrating harder on keeping your knees apart and using your buttock muscles to push up to standing, and your thigh muscles when you are lowering yourself into sitting.

Maximum 40: progress by holding onto weights.

This exercise is helpful in strengthening your legs and keeping your hip and knee joints lubricated and healthy.

Chin ins

Sit against the back of the chair. Poke your chin forward as if you are crossing a finishing line at a race. Now take your chin back as if you are being force-fed something you don't want. Ensure that you are looking straight ahead and not up or down.

Maximum 10

This exercise is good for flexibility and strength of your neck muscles.

Tummy tucks

Get onto your hands and knees. Lift up the part just below your belly button and hold while you breathe in and out three times. It's not easy but try and persist. If you find it difficult to kneel on the floor, try the exercise on your bed or a firm sofa.

Maximum 10

This exercise targets your core stabilisers or the deep muscles in your lower back and stomach area.

Back arches

Lie on your stomach and place your hands near your shoulders. Push up and arch your back, keeping your lower body flat on the floor.

Maximum 10

This exercise helps strengthen your arms and increases the flexibility of your back.

	Sit-ups Lie on your back with your knees bent upwards (crook lying position). Curl your upper body into a crunch. You can rest your hands on your stomach or slide your hands along your thighs towards your knees as you curl. Pick a point in the ceiling and focus on it to keep your neck still. Don't bend your neck towards your knees as you complete the sit-up. *Maximum 30* *This exercise helps strengthen your abdominal muscles.*
	Scissor legs Lie on your side with your head resting on a pillow or cushion. Lift your leg straight up to the side. Make sure that you are not moving your leg forward or behind you. *Maximum 10: progress by placing a small weight around the ankle.* *This exercise helps strengthen your hip and buttock muscles.*

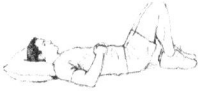

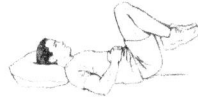

Tuck-ins

Lie on your back and bend your knees and while keeping your feet flat on the ground. Place your hands on your stomach. Without using your hands, raise your feet off the floor and bring your knees towards your chest and back down again.

Maximum 20: progress by straightening your legs out slowly in a gentle arc as you put your feet down.

This exercise helps to strengthen your hip flexors and core stabilisers.

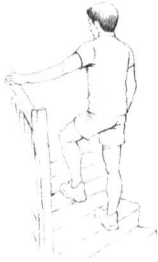

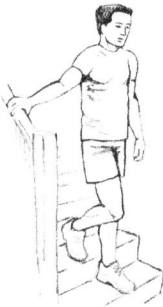

Stairs

Find some stairs. Climb the stairs as you would if you were pain free – one foot on one step, the other foot on the step above. Avoid climbing and leading with the same foot. Also avoid going up or down sideways. However many steps you walk up, you need to walk down. If you walk up five and then walk down those five, it is counted as five steps.

Maximum 30: progress by going faster or holding weights.

This exercise strengthens your bones, muscles, ligaments and keeps your joints lubricated and healthy.

Shoulder press

Take a manageable weight in your hands, while standing with your feet comfortably apart. If you don't have weights use a tin of soup or a bottle of water. Look straight ahead and raise the weight above your head as far as you can manage. Bring one arm down and raise the other one. Do this slowly.

Maximum 20: progress by increasing the weight.

This exercise helps to strengthen your neck, shoulder and arm muscles.

Jogging

There are three levels at which you can do this exercise. The first level is where you are jogging on the spot, only raising your feet slightly off the floor with little bend at your knees. The next level is when you raise your feet with more bend at your knees. The third level is when you are actually jogging. Start at the level with which you feel comfortable. In the beginning you might only be able to manage 30 seconds. That is okay, so long as you gradually increase each week.

Maximum 10 minutes: progress by running faster.

This exercise will improve your leg strength, endurance and fitness.

Once you've tried all of the exercises and have set your start points, it's time to begin your first week of exercising.

Remember to keep to the numbers you've set. Try your best and know that you are on your way to feeling better, fitter and stronger.

Of course, if there is an exercise you simply cannot do now, then leave it and revisit it in a week or two.

USING REFLECTION AND PACING UP

Look at the numbers you have achieved for all the exercises. Reflect on how manageable they were. If you did five sit-ups and had some difficulty with them, have a think about how many you could do in the second week of exercise. You might feel that you could manage six sit-ups. If you did them fairly easily, you may pace up the amount to seven or eight sit-ups to do in the second week.

At the end of the first week, each of the exercises requires this careful consideration. As you become familiar with them, you will do this weekly reflection more quickly.

Don't forget that it is important to only ever increase the numbers, not decrease. In other words, don't go from five sit-ups in one week to eight in the next week before you're ready, then decide that eight are too many and go back to five the week after. It's better to go from five to six, and then maybe seven or eight when you are ready. Pacing up the amounts weekly will work best. Remember that pacing up needs to be a gradual increase in the amounts you do.

It is vital for you to start slowly and comfortably pace up your exercises until you reach the repetition limits.

At the end of the first week:

1. For each exercise, carefully consider what you feel you can comfortably pace up for the second week. If you are unsure, increase by 20-25%.
2. Choose three days during the week to do the exercises and fill in the numbers on your chart. The days can change from week to week.

3. Have a look to see if you think your numbers are manageable. Remember, once you set your new week's numbers, like in the example below, you need to stick to them.

4. Avoid the overactivity–underactivity rollercoaster. Be conservative and pace up faster the following week if you are finding it too easy. Your plan for week 2 might look like this:

	Week 1 of exercise					Week 2 of exercise				
	Mon	Tues	Wed	Thurs	Fri	Mon	Tues	Wed	Thurs	Fri
Arm Circles (max 2 mins)	20 secs ✓	Break	20 secs ✓	Break	20 secs ✓	30 secs	30 secs	Break	30 secs	Break
Side Leans (max 10)	3 ✓	Break	3 ✓	Break	3 ✓	4	4	Break	4	Break
Lunge Squats (max 15)	2 ✓	Break	2 ✓	Break	2 ✓	5	5	Break	5	Break

The grid above shows how the numbers are filled in for week 2 before the exercises have been done. When the exercises are completed each day, tick them off to acknowledge that they have been done.

It doesn't matter how fast or how slowly you increase your numbers, just as long as you do increase them. Your increases don't have to be consistent. In the first week, you might do two lunge squats then increase to five in the second week, then you might find this is harder and decide you'll only increase the number of lunge squats to six in the third week. Even though you increased by three in week 2, and only by one in week 3, you are still pacing up. Remember the key is to never decrease. Be conservative and don't set yourself up to fail.

You may find some exercises are easier than others. If

this is the case, it's also okay to pace up different exercises at different rates. For example, as shown below, you may increase side leans by one every week because you find them difficult, but increase another easier exercise by several more repetitions.

	Week 1 of exercise					Week 2 of exercise					Week 3 of exercise				
	Mon	Tues	Wed	Thurs	Fri	Mon	Tues	Wed	Thurs	Fri	Mon	Tues	Wed	Thurs	Fri
Arm Circles (max 2 mins)	20 secs ✓	Break	20 secs ✓	Break ✓	20 secs	30 secs ✓	30 secs ✓	Break	30 secs ✓	Break	35 secs	Break	35 secs	Break	35 secs
Side Leans (max 10)	3 ✓	Break	3 ✓	Break ✓	3	4 ✓	4 ✓	Break	4 ✓	Break	6	Break	6	Break	6
Lunge Squats (max 15)	2 ✓	Break	2 ✓	Break ✓	2	5 ✓	5 ✓	Break	5 ✓	Break	6	Break	6	Break	6

The exercise program video can be viewed for free by scanning the QR code, or by visiting www.beyondpain.com.au and navigating to the 'Downloads' page.

MAKING THE EXERCISES MORE CHALLENGING

Once you are comfortably managing the maximum number of a particular exercise, you can further challenge yourself by adding weights, increasing the speed of that exercise or by replacing that exercise with a more difficult exercise. Make a note of the changes to your plan and set new start points.

If you add weights to your exercises, you might need to lower your repetitions. For example, if you did the maximum amount of 20 shoulder presses with 1 kg dumbbells comfortably, and then you want to increase to 2 kg dumbbells, you might drop back to 10 shoulder presses and build up again. Have a try and decide what is manageable for you, use this as a starting point and then pace up. This is not going backwards, because you are actually making the exercise harder even though you are doing fewer repetitions.

Instead of adding weights, you might want to pace up by doing an activity faster. For example, you may want to walk to the shops faster, ride your bike to work faster or perhaps jog around the park faster. In these cases you need to pace up by actually reducing the time to cover the distance week after week. For example, if it took you fifteen minutes to walk to the shops in week 1, you might decide to do it in thirteen minutes in week 2.

No matter how you modify your exercises, or what new exercises you decide to do, you need to set new starting points and pace up each week. Pacing yourself will take the struggle out of achieving your goals, and make the experience more enjoyable.

NOT A FAN OF EXERCISE PROGRAMS?

If you are not a fan of exercise programs, use this program as a platform to get your strength and endurance back to do the things you really enjoy doing. You are not expected to do these forever, but in the shorter term, they will help get your fitness back. And the more you do, the more you will be able to do. Remember, once you get back to your enjoyable activities, then you no longer need to continue with this exercise program. Your enjoyable activities should provide you with the exercise.

Exercise plan – example

	Week __ of exercise					Week __ of exercise					Week __ of exercise				
	Mon	Tues	Wed	Thurs	Fri	Mon	Tues	Wed	Thurs	Fri	Mon	Tues	Wed	Thurs	Fri
Arm Circles Max 2mins or 40 circles	20 secs ✓	Break	20 secs ✓	Break	20 secs ✓	30 secs ✓	30 secs ✓	Break	30 secs ✓	Break	35 secs	Break	35 secs	Break	35 secs
Side Leans (max 10)	3 ✓	Break	3 ✓	Break	3 ✓	4 ✓	4 ✓	Break	4 ✓	Break	6	Break	6	Break	6
Lunge Squats (max 15)	2 ✓	Break	2 ✓	Break	2 ✓	5 ✓	5 ✓	Break	5	Break	6	Break	6	Break	6
Sit to Stands Max 40	12 ✓	Break	12 ✓	Break	12 ✓	15 ✓	15 ✓	Break	15 ✓	Break	20	Break	20	Break	20
Chin Ins Max 10	10 ✓	Break	10 ✓	Break	10 ✓	10 ✓	10 ✓	Break	10 ✓	Break	10	Break	10	Break	10
Tummy Tucks Max 10	10 ✓	Break	10 ✓	Break	10 ✓	10 ✓	10 ✓	Break	10 ✓	Break	10	Break	10	Break	10
Back Arches Max10	8 ✓	Break	8 ✓	Break	8 ✓	10 ✓	10 ✓	Break	10 ✓	Break	10	Break	10	Break	10
Sit Ups Max 30	4 ✓	Break	4 ✓	Break	4 ✓	6 ✓	6 ✓	Break	6 ✓	Break	10	Break	10	Break	10
Scissor Legs Max10	5 ✓	Break	5 ✓	Break	5 ✓	6 ✓	6 ✓	Break	6 ✓	Break	7	Break	7	Break	7
Tuck Ins Max 20	10 ✓	Break	10 ✓	Break	10 ✓	12 ✓	12 ✓	Break	12 ✓	Break	16	Break	16	Break	16
Stairs/ Steps Max 30 steps	10 ✓	Break	10 ✓	Break	10 ✓	13 ✓	13 ✓	Break	13 ✓	Break	18	Break	18	Break	18
Shoulder Presses Max 20	12 ✓	Break	12 ✓	Break	12 ✓	14 ✓	14 ✓	Break	14 ✓	Break	16	Break	16	Break	16
Jogging Max 10 Mins	2 ✓	Break	2 ✓	Break	2 ✓	5 ✓	5 ✓	Break	5 ✓	Break	8	Break	8	Break	8
Optional own Exercise															

Weekly review

- Fill in the plan for your exercises.
- Start your exercises and remember to tick them off once you've completed them.
- Complete the exercises program three times a week.
- At the end of the week, reflect on your exercise plan and set new numbers for the following week. Remember to pace up the numbers.

And continue...

- Building on your daily activities.
- Being aware of your body and focusing on the gains.
- Pacing to an amount or time, not pain.
- Doing daily warm-ups and stretches.
- Repeating your affirmations and affirmation questions.
- Doing a weekly planner for the week ahead. Remember to review your weekly planner to identify any patterns. Rejoice any achievements.
- Reflecting on the goals you set to ensure that they are still achievable. Change them if you need to. See how you can use your exercises to help build your strength and flexibility to help achieve them.

WEEK 4

THE RIGHT MINDSET

Now that you have set your goals, started your stretching and exercise programs, and begun to feel better, it's time to reflect on your thinking. For this program to work at its best, the changes you are making need to be both physical and psychological.

Now that your body is showing you that it can manage things you never thought you could, you have to change your perceptions of yourself. Rewrite your truths. Your body believes what your mind tells it, so now you have to start telling it something different. A couple of weeks ago, you might have told yourself: *I can't...* whereas now, you need to start telling yourself: *I can...*

A right mindset is not fearing pain or trying to avoid it, but looking towards the future and knowing that you can deal with whatever pain levels you may experience.

CHALLENGING UNHELPFUL THOUGHTS

Replace your unhelpful thoughts with more helpful ones that will serve you better. This will put you in a more positive frame of mind. Remember those traffic lights on the pain highway? Helpful thoughts and attitudes keep them red; unhelpful thoughts keep them green.

Changing thoughts

Try changing unhelpful thoughts into helpful thoughts:

Why can't I just get rid of this pain?	becomes	At least I am walking more now and I can get out of the house.
I hate my pain.	becomes	The pain is frustrating but if I continue to pace myself, I'll be able to do this.
This pain is controlling my life.	becomes	I'm not going to put my life on hold for this.
I can't live like this.	becomes	This is something I will learn to manage and live with.
I should push through the pain.	becomes	I could pace myself and slowly build up my tolerances.
I should avoid things that make my pain worse.	becomes	I'm not going to limit myself. If my pain does increase, I will learn to manage it.

We already know that your thoughts can affect how your body responds. If you make sure your thinking is helpful, you end up in a positive frame of mind. It might sound false at first, but the research doesn't lie.

If you recognise yourself saying some of the negative things above, here are a few strategies that can pull you out of that kind of thinking.

The four questions

This activity is quick and easy and involves asking yourself these questions:

- Is it *fair* to be so critical of yourself?
- Is it *true* what you are saying about you or your situation? Where is the proof?
- Is it *helpful* for you to think along these lines?
- If you heard your best friend saying these things, what would you say to encourage them?

Changing from 'I should' to 'I could'

You may blame yourself during times of increased pain. You may have thoughts such as:

- I should have done this.
- I should have stopped earlier.

Try changing these to more helpful statements:

- I could have done it this way.
- I could stop earlier next time.

Changing from 'I can't' to 'I can'

When your confidence is low or you start to fear your pain, you may have thoughts such as:

- I can't do that.
- I can't possibly kneel on the floor to play with the kids.

These *I can't* statements put you in a negative frame of mind. Instead of thinking about what you *can't* do, think about what you *can* do:

- I can try this.
- I can try kneeling on a cushion as a start and slowly make progress.

Some people avoid the things that they enjoy because of their negative mindset. They don't play golf, play with the grandkids, work in the garden or play sport because they fear that they may end up in more pain. In the quest to avoid pain, they get into a cycle of inactivity and end up in more pain.

Being unfit, inactive and frustrated because you are missing out on many of the enjoyable things life has to offer makes you susceptible to higher pain levels.

Don't fear chronic pain. The best attitude is accepting that you have pain, accepting that there will be times of increased pain no matter what you do, and know that you will successfully manage it.

Try the following strategies and find what works best for you.

Worksheets can be found at the back of this book, by scanning the QR code, or by visiting www.beyondpain.com.au and navigating to the 'Downloads' page.

PERSPECTIVE

A strategy that has helped a lot of people to change their unhelpful thinking is to put things into perspective. You might think your situation is bad until you meet someone whose situation is so much worse than yours that you almost feel ashamed for giving your own situation so much importance. Don't feel ashamed and don't wait until someone offers you a comparison. Come up with your own comparisons.

Perspective scale

Think of your own scale of bad things that could happen. It may look like this:

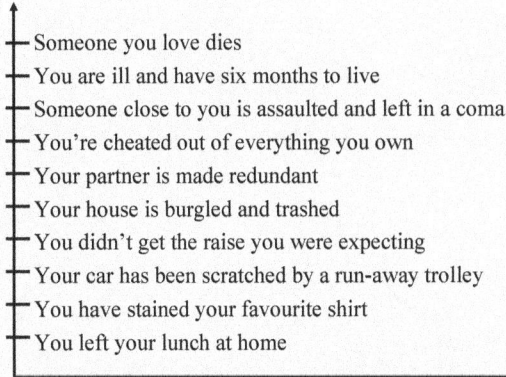

- Someone you love dies
- You are ill and have six months to live
- Someone close to you is assaulted and left in a coma
- You're cheated out of everything you own
- Your partner is made redundant
- Your house is burgled and trashed
- You didn't get the raise you were expecting
- Your car has been scratched by a run-away trolley
- You have stained your favourite shirt
- You left your lunch at home

Imagine that you weren't able to complete your shopping because of your pain and you are angry and upset that you can't even get a simple task done. You think that *things just can't get any worse*.

But where would you put your situation on your perspective scale?

Keep a copy of the scale with you and when you are in an unhelpful frame of mind, place your situation on this scale. It might be worse than forgetting your lunch, but it probably isn't as bad as your partner being made redundant.

Keeping a copy of your perspective scale in your handbag or wallet can be handy because it doesn't involve a lot of thought. When you're feeling upset with your pain, read the list and see that it's not as bad as you may think.

Another effective strategy to manage unhelpful thoughts is to use a Thoughts Challenger sheet. Often during times of difficulty, so many thoughts and feelings go through our heads that there are too many to remember. The idea behind the Thoughts Challenger sheet is to get all your thoughts and emotions on paper, challenge the unhelpful ones using the strategies we have discussed, and then replace these with more helpful thoughts. Often, people find it is easier to have each unhelpful thought written down and then challenge them individually. It gives them time to reflect.

Thoughts Challenger Sheet

- Think of a situation that has put you in a negative frame of mind.
- Fill in the three headings like the example.
- Ask yourself the four questions below.
- Fill in the three columns

Situation	Initial thoughts	Initial emotions
Couldn't finish vacuuming the whole house	*I am useless* *Why can't I do this* *I will never be able to do this*	Anger, frustration, helplessness

↓

Challenge your thoughts

The four questions

- Is it true?
- Is it helpful?
- Is it fair?
- What would you say to your best friend to encourage them if they were in your shoes?

Or ask an affirmation question:

- Why will I be able to finish vacuuming the whole house in the future?
- Why can I now do some of the vacuuming?

↓

More helpful thoughts	New emotions	Helpful behaviour and an action plan
I have done half of the vacuuming. Before starting this program I couldn't do any of it. *Or: It's better to pace. It doesn't really matter if I leave some of the vacuuming for another day.*	Some disappointment but calmer, happier, a sense of achievement rather than failure	Change to something different now. Refer to this sheet if similar feelings occur during the similar situation. Continue to pace activities. Use management strategies before, during and after the activity.

Look at your unhelpful thoughts and think of how you can turn them into more helpful thoughts. It may be that instead of thinking *I am useless,* you think *I may not be able to do what I want, but I have made a start on...*

If you have difficulty coming up with helpful thoughts, think about how you want to feel in the situation, maybe less stressed or less angry, and ask yourself what thoughts would you need to feel this way.

The Thoughts Challenger sheet aims to help you see a situation in a more helpful way. I don't expect you to use a Thoughts Challenger sheet for every difficult situation, but if you use it regularly and form the habit of challenging unhelpful thinking, this process will become automatic. It's all about thinking I can... I will... why will I be able to?

Weekly review

- Fill in the Thoughts Challenger sheet for two difficult situations that you encounter during the week. If you don't experience two situations, think about a time when you had a pain flare-up, use this situation as practice for using the Thoughts Challenger sheet.
- Make your own bad situations scale and use it on one occasion during the week.
- Consciously include *I can... I will... I could...* statements in your thinking.

And continue...

- Building on your daily activities.
- Being aware of your body and focusing on the gains.
- Pacing to an amount or time, not pain.
- Doing daily warm-ups and stretches.
- Exercising three times a week.
- Filling in your exercise plan for the following week, remembering to increase the numbers.
- Repeating your affirmations and affirmation questions.
- Doing a weekly planner for the week ahead. Remember to review your weekly planner to identify any patterns. Rejoice any achievements.
- Working on your goals. Remember, this is the bigger picture.

WEEK 5

PUTTING JOY BACK INTO YOUR LIFE

If you suffer from pain, finding joy and fun in your life might be the very last thing on your mind. But as we have seen throughout this book, these things are important because they take the focus away from your pain.

If you haven't already done so, look back at your goals and see if you can make a start on them. Remember that having fun and being joyful releases endorphins that help turn the lights on the pain highway to red, blocking the pain messages.

ACTIVITY-RELAX CYCLES

You should be familiar with activity-relax cycles. Now incorporate them into your enjoyable activities. As with your daily activities, ensure that you don't overdo the things you enjoy and think about a manageable amount for you. Just say that you want to play a game with your kids at the park. You might find that you can play with them for ten minutes and then you need to relax for ten minutes. That is okay.

Write down your activity-relax cycles for your enjoyable activities in your journal so that you can track progress.

Remember that your activity-relax cycles need to have a combination of both activity and relaxation. Remember that the relaxation period does not mean that you have to be inactive; it can be something less active. For example, if your *activity* was kicking a ball at the park with your kids, then your *relaxation* period might be leaving the game to help with the barbecue or reading a magazine while they play. If your activity was jogging for fifteen minutes, your relaxation period could be walking at a gentle pace for five minutes.

As with pacing your day-to-day activities, don't get caught into doing something active like gardening and then deciding that your relaxation period should be cleaning the gutters. Can you see that both of these require you to be physically active? The reverse is also true. If you are playing on the computer, your *relaxation* period doesn't mean you should go sit on the couch and watch TV. Also, be mindful of your body's natural painkillers masking your pain.

Ensure that you start conservatively. It is all in the pacing.

Remember that using the activity-relax cycle will allow you to achieve your goals in a more enjoyable, rewarding way. In turn, it will also give you the confidence that you *can* do it.

BEING CREATIVE

You can be creative when you are pacing up your goals and activities; you don't need to just pace time. If it is your desire to dance to songs on the radio, then you can pace up your dancing by increasing the number of songs you dance to in a row each week. If you want to kick a football at the park with your kids, you might pace up by the number of times you can kick the ball during each park visit. If your desire is to get back into the kitchen and cook for your family, you can build up the number of meals you cook each week, or you can increase the complexity and the amount of time it takes to cook a meal – go from toast to a roast.

Always aim to improve and increase the amounts. Use whatever measures you like to show the improvement.

Pacing up of activities

The plan below shows a mother with chronic knee pain whose goal it is to spend more time playing on the floor with her young children. She wants to do this each day. In the first week, she has chosen a manageable amount. Once she feels comfortable with the ten minutes each morning, she aims to increase it to two short periods each day. In the third week, she is aiming for three short periods each day.

Monday:	10 minutes: morning
Tuesday:	10 minutes: morning
Wednesday:	10 minutes: morning
Thursday:	10 minutes: morning
Friday:	10 minutes: morning
Saturday:	10 minutes: morning
Sunday:	10 minutes: morning
Monday:	10 minutes: morning and afternoon
Tuesday:	10 minutes: morning and afternoon
Wednesday:	10 minutes: morning and afternoon
Thursday:	10 minutes: morning and afternoon
Friday:	10 minutes: morning and afternoon
Saturday:	10 minutes: morning and afternoon
Sunday:	10 minutes: morning and afternoon
Monday:	10 minutes: morning and afternoon , and evening
Tuesday:	10 minutes: morning and afternoon , and evening
Wednesday:	10 minutes: morning and afternoon , and evening
Thursday:	10 minutes: morning and afternoon , and evening
Friday:	10 minutes: morning and afternoon , and evening
Saturday:	10 minutes: morning and afternoon , and evening
Sunday:	10 minutes: morning and afternoon , and evening

If you enjoy dancing and your goal is to go out with friends to a dance club, pace up a few weeks before the event. Decide how much you can manage and then increase that amount. You could choose to measure your progress by counting how many consecutive songs you dance to. You could start by dancing to two songs, twice a week and then build up. Your logbook might look something like this:

Week 1	Two songs, twice a week
Week 2	Three songs, twice a week
Week 3	Four songs, twice a week
Week 4	Five songs, twice a week
Week 5	Six songs, twice a week

It is common for people with chronic pain to use heat or ice to distract their brain from the pain. The use of heat and ice can be incorporated into pacing. For example, people often say that they feel better after a hot shower in the morning, or that putting ice on their painful joints at the end of the day takes the edge off their pain.

One of my young clients was a keen basketball player and used to routinely have fifteen minutes of court time and then sit out for five minutes with an ice-pack on his painful right knee (even when his knee was feeling good). Then he would return to the game for another fifteen minutes. He gradually built up his court time to be able to play a full game, and used an ice-pack for five minutes after the game. He iced his knee post match routinely irrespective of how good or bad his knee was. This helped him manage his pain, and more importantly, allowed him to do what he enjoyed.

NOT MISSING OUT

Every now and then, you might get the opportunity to do something that you know will cause a flare-up of your pain, but you don't want to miss out. You might have bought tickets to a concert of your favourite rock band, been invited to the football grand-final, or friends are going to a long movie that you've been waiting to see for ages. You say 'yes' because it's something you really want to do, even though you know you will probably suffer the next day. It is kind of like when we have a night out on the town partying; we know we're going to feel rotten the next morning, but it's worth it!

Even though you know there will be pain consequences, there are ways to lessen them; it is about what you can do before, during and after the event.

The three Ps:

$P = Prioritise$
$P = Plan$
$P = Pace$

- *Prioritise*

If you're going to a concert on Saturday night, you need to prioritise your activities before, during and after the concert. Your stretches and exercises are a priority because they will be important to help you feel good before the concert. You may have planned to go shopping on the same day, but you need to do this on another day. You need to prioritise what is important on the day of the activity so that you don't overdo things.

- *Plan*

Do your stretches on Saturday morning.

Exercises after lunch.

Rest or relax in the afternoon.

Concert in the evening – pace while you are there.

Gentle stretches when you get home.

Gentle stretches the next morning.

- *Pace*

Relax and feel good about your choice to go to the concert.

Take the time to change positions regularly when you are at the concert.

Move around if you can.

If *I can't* thoughts creep in *(I can't do this; I can't last the whole concert)*, challenge them with *I can* thoughts *(I can last for the next set of songs; I can move around and stretch a bit)*.

KEEPING TRACK

So far you have learned some very important strategies for the management of your pain. You have practiced these strategies weekly and should now be working towards achieving your goals.

To help implement these strategies into your goals, create a table in your logbook to keep track of how you are implementing the strategies.

The following table can be found at the back of this book, by scanning the QR code, or by visiting www.beyondpain.com.au and navigating to the 'Downloads' page.

Your table might look like this:

Week	Strategy	Goal 1	Goal 2
		Bush walking for one hour in one month	Cleaning the whole house in two months' time.
1	Affirmations	I will manage to walk each day for longer periods. I will pace myself and keep my pain at bay.	I will manage to clean two rooms each week. I will make sure I am not struggling.
	Activity-relax cycle	I will pace my daily activities so that I have enough energy to do my bush walk.	I will pace my daily activities for the rest of the day so that I don't collapse in the evening.
	Journal	I will record what went well and what didn't. I will write my feelings and think about what I can do better next time.	I will record what went well and what didn't. I will write my feelings and think about what I can do better next time.
2	Goal Setting	I have set a realistic goal of bush walking for an hour and I plan to practice once a week	I have set a realistic goal of cleaning the house, and I will start by cleaning for just 30 minutes three times per week.

	Affirmation questions	Why will I be able to bush walk for an hour? Why will it be more enjoyable?	Why will I clean the house without too much pain? Why will I enjoy it more this time?
	Stretch Program	I will do my stretch program before and after my bush walk to help manage my symptoms.	I will do my stretch program before my cleaning to help manage my symptoms.
3	Exercises	I will do the exercises on alternative days so that I don't have too much on.	I will do the exercises later in the evening to break up my day.
4	Challenging thoughts	I have done a thoughts challenger sheet to challenge my unhelpful thinking.	I have done a thoughts challenger sheet to challenge my unhelpful thinking.
5	Enjoyable Activities	I will use an activity-relax cycle by walking for 20 minutes then having a break or five minutes to either do a few stretches or just stop and enjoy the scenery.	I will use an activity-relax cycle by vacuuming for 10 minutes then doing some light dusting for five minutes. After one room, I will have a cup of tea to break things up.
6	Relaxation techniques	I will do at least five quick relaxes as I walk. I might use a visualisation session after lunch, and use an auditory distraction technique or two at some point during my walk.	I will use quick relaxes as I vacuum. Afterwards I will do a visualisation session.
7	Improving sleep	I will ensure I prepare myself for a good night's sleep the night before my walk.	I will ensure that I get to bed early the night before and pace myself so that I can sleep well on the day.
8	Flare-up and setbacks: problem-solving plan	I will develop a problem-solving plan in case I do experience difficulties.	I will develop a problem-solving plan in case I do experience difficulties.

Weekly review

- Focus on enjoyable activities.
- Develop a plan to do a number of enjoyable activities. Remember to consider the activity-relax cycle. Make a note of your progress in your logbook.
- Complete a tracking sheet for two of your goals.
- Try pacing up one of the enjoyable activities in a creative way like dancing to one song, then two.
- Reflect on the goals and apply some of these pacing principles to them. For example, you may incorporate an activity-rest cycle into one of your goals.

And continue...

- Building on your daily activities.
- Being aware of your body and focusing on the gains.
- Pacing to an amount or time, not pain.
- Doing daily warm-ups and stretches.
- Exercising three times a week.
- Filling in your exercise plan for the following week, and remembering to pace up the numbers.
- Repeating your affirmations and affirmation questions.
- Doing a weekly planner for the week ahead. Remember to review your weekly planner to identify any patterns. Rejoice any achievements.
- Using the Thoughts Challenger sheet so that you become more familiar with challenging unhelpful thinking. If you encounter any hurdles use it, otherwise think of situations that it may be useful for, and practice.

WEEK 6

RELAXATION TECHNIQUES

By now you will feel a lot fitter, more energetic, more flexible, and be in a happier more positive frame of mind. Now it is time to learn some relaxation techniques to assist you in further managing your pain levels.

Relaxation techniques help ease anxiety, worry and tension in your body. Relaxation also helps clear your mind and even makes your body feel lighter. A clearer mind and a lighter body mean less focus on your pain. People often use relaxation sessions before going to bed to help rid their mind of the day's thoughts and worries. A relaxed mind means a better night's sleep.

There are several types of relaxation techniques. Some can be done quickly and easily to take the edge off your pain when you are stuck in a traffic jam or on a crowded train, while others require you to focus on an object or sound when you are in a comfortable place and have a bit of time to spare. They are all useful.

Before you learn the relaxation techniques, you need to learn how to breathe deeply. Deep breathing helps reduce pain and muscle tension, and combined with relaxation techniques, forms an effective strategy for managing pain, anxiety and muscle tension.

DEEP BREATHING

Deep breathing in a relaxed manner allows air to get into the base of your lungs. To feel the difference between deep breathing and regular breathing is simple. With deep breathing, when you breathe in, your stomach will rise along with your chest. When you breathe out, both go down.

This is referred to as breathing through your diaphragm. When you are breathing normally, just your chest moves in and out, not your stomach. To practice:

1. Get yourself into a comfortable position – ideally lying down on your back with your knees bent and feet flat on the ground, or lying on your side. If lying is difficult, sit in a comfortable seat.
2. Rest your hands on your stomach so that you can feel your stomach rise and fall.
3. Breathe in and focus on your stomach pushing out in a slow, relaxed manner.
4. Pause for a second.
5. Breathe out slowly and feel your stomach go back down.
6. As you breathe out, let your body totally relax and create a sense of letting go.
7. Continue to breathe normally but in a relaxed manner.

If you got it first time, great. If not, just practice, you will get it.

 A video on how to deep breathe can be viewed for free by scanning the QR code, or by visiting www.beyondpain.com.au and navigating to the 'Downloads' page.

THREE TYPES OF RELAXATION TECHNIQUES

- Quick relaxes: As the name suggests, these are quick and easy and will take you about a minute or so to do. They consist of relaxed deep breathing, and can be done throughout the day to take the edge off anxiety, and stop the build-up of tension.
- Distraction techniques: These take around five minutes, and encourage you to focus on a sound or object to distract you from your pain.

- Visualisation techniques: These take around 20 minutes. You create a quiet calm place in your mind, and then enter the place by picturing yourself among the calm.

Audio instructions for various relaxation techniques can be listened to for free by scanning the QR code, or by visiting www.beyondpain.com.au and navigating to the 'Downloads' page.

QUICK RELAXES

These are very effective when you need to take the edge off your pain. They take only around a minute. Quick relaxes can be done while walking, standing, lying down or sitting up. They can be done when you are squashed on a crowded train, or stuck in a traffic jam. You can also use them when dancing, walking the dog, or watching TV. Here are three types of quick relaxes. Choose one that suits you best.

Wave of relaxation	Take a deep breath in, pause for a moment, and say the word *relax* to yourself as you breathe out.
	Continue to breathe in and out in a slow, relaxed way.
	As you do this, imagine a wave of relaxation flowing down from your forehead, to your face, and down to your neck and shoulders.
	As the wave flows down, relax any excess tension in your neck and shoulders.
	Now, feel the wave of relaxation flowing down your arms, to your hands and out through your fingertips, taking away any excess tension.
	Take a deep breath in again, pause and then breathe out. Continue to breathe in a nice relaxed way
	Feel the wave of relaxation now running down your chest, to your stomach and to your back muscles.
	Relax any excess tension in your back.

Now, feel the wave of relaxation going down into your buttocks, your thighs, and down into your feet.

Feel the wave flowing out through your toes taking away any excess tension.

Take a deep breath in, pause and say the word *relax* to yourself as you breathe out.

One word, one breath

Think of a word that will help you to relax. It may be the word *peace, calm, safe* or simply *relax*.

Take a deep breath in, hold for a moment, and then repeat the word in a gentle slow-paced manner as you breathe out.

Count down

This quick-relax is particularly helpful when you are performing an activity such as walking up a hill or cycling.

Imagine the number 10 in your mind, and say the word *relax* in a calm soothing manner.

Now imagine the number 9, and say the word *relax* in a calm soothing manner.

Continue this until you count down to 1.

Once you have done this, take a deep breath in, pause, and say the word *relax* to yourself as you breathe out.

Signs that you might need to incorporate quick relaxes into your daily routine are increases in: muscle tension, pain, muscle spasms, anxiety, stress, anger or frustration.

If you incorporate quick relaxes into your daily routine, they will help you to prevent a build-up of pain and muscle tension. Try doing quick relaxes in ad breaks when you are watching TV, before and after meals, when you are having a break at work, when you are stuck in traffic. You can also do them while running, walking, or doing your exercises and stretches.

People who use these techniques many times a day find them very helpful because they relieve small amounts of tension throughout the day. By the end of the day, they feel less tired and have less pain.

DISTRACTION TECHNIQUES

There are two useful ways to combine relaxation and distraction to manage your pain. These can also be used if you are stuck in a frustrating situation like being stuck on a plane or taxi. You can focus on either an object or a sound.

Focusing on an object

Do a quick-relax technique first to get yourself into a more relaxed state.

Choose an object in front of you. It can be a painting, an antique clock or a car parked on the street.

Concentrate on what the object looks like. What shape is it? What are the contours like?

Concentrate on the colour.

Concentrate on what you see.

Keep your focus for around five minutes.

Focusing on a sound

Do a quick-relax technique first to get yourself into a more relaxed state.

Listen to some instrumental or relaxation music, or listen to a sound such as a heater, an air-conditioner or the traffic outside.

Concentrate on the sound.

Concentrate on what you hear. How loud is it? How deep or soft is it? What is the rhythm or beat like?

Immerse yourself in the sound.

Keep your focus for around five minutes.

VISUALISATION

Visualisation is a longer and deeper version of relaxation. It is very effective and should be practised once or twice a day. Visualisation goes hand in hand with the quick relaxes and distraction techniques; none are replacements for each other. Practising all types of relaxation regularly will help you the most. With practice, your body will relax on cue.

This technique involves visualising a relaxing or calming scene – it may be somewhere you have been in the past, somewhere you want to go, or somewhere imaginary. Some people find it easier to visualise an activity such as snorkelling around coral reefs or fishing in a calm lake. Whatever you choose, you need to have a sense of peace and relaxation when you think of this scene.

The key is to be in the scene, as opposed to being a person looking at the scene. You need to imagine what you would see, feel, hear and smell as if you were actually there.

Find a quiet place that allows you to relax.

1. Get into a comfortable position

   Pause for 20 seconds.

2. Take a long slow breath in, pause at the top of the breath, and say the word relax as you exhale. Allow yourself to feel a sensation of relaxation as you continue to breathe in a relaxed manner. Allow your forehead to relax, allow your face and your jaw to relax, and then allow your neck and shoulders to relax. Feel the sensation of heaviness flow downwards to your arms, hands and out through your fingertips. As you continue to breathe in a relaxed manner, feel the relaxation flowing down your chest, your back, and your buttocks. Feel the sense of heaviness flowing down your thighs, feet and out through your toes.

   Pause for 10 seconds.

3. Now imagine that you are in your peaceful place.

   Pause for 60 seconds.

4. Take a moment to imagine what you *see* in your peaceful place. Look around in all directions. What do you see around you? Behind you? Imagine what the quality of light is like. Take a moment to focus on what you see.

    Pause for 60 seconds.

5. Now focus on what you *hear* in your peaceful place. Focus on all the different sounds that you hear: waves, leaves rustling, a gentle breeze, birds chirping or crackling firewood.

    Pause for 60 seconds.

6. Now focus on what you *feel* in your peaceful place. Is it warm, mild or cool? Can you feel the wind blowing or the sun shining on your body? Take a moment to focus on what you feel in this pleasant and peaceful place.

    Pause for 60 seconds.

7. Focus on the smells in your peaceful place: the salty sea breeze, fresh-cut grass or flowers.

    Pause for 60 seconds.

8. Now focus on any pleasant *tastes* in your peaceful place. Are you having a cool or warm drink? Are you eating something delicious? Savour any pleasant tastes that are present.

    Pause for 60 seconds

9. Spend a few minutes just being in your peaceful place and enjoy your pleasant and relaxing scene.

    Pause 3-5 minutes.

10. When you feel ready, begin to think of opening your eyes. Let this happen slowly as you count backwards from 10 to 1.

    As you are counting to yourself 10... 9... 8... notice how calmly you are breathing.

    Slowly open your eyes during the countdown and allow your eyes to adjust to the light.

    Notice how your mind and body are now relaxed.

412   BEYOND PAIN

There are times, however, when unpleasant thoughts and images may come to mind when you do this technique. When this happens, imagine those thoughts and images are like clouds passing by to give you a clear blue sky.

If you find that your pain is distracting you, take a step back and try and recreate the atmosphere, go back into the detail and try to absorb yourself back into the scene.

Following each session, take the time to reflect on how it was. Was the relaxation experience enjoyable? How did it make you feel? Don't reflect on simply whether the relaxation technique made your pain go away. You will notice that the more you relax, the less muscle tension you will have, and that this leads to a decrease in the pain you feel.

Relaxation techniques take practice. Keep working at them until they come naturally and easily.

Weekly review

- Build up to five quick relaxes per day. Try different ones to see what works for you best. Try them at different times – before, during or after activities. Write the most helpful ones in your logbook.
- Try one of the distraction techniques.
- Try a visualisation technique.
- Review your logbook. Try and identify patterns in the times you feel increases or decreases in pain. What strategies are working for you?

And continue...

- Building on your daily activities.
- Being aware of your body and focusing on the gains.
- Pacing to an amount or time, not pain.
- Doing daily warm-ups and stretches.
- Exercising three times a week.

- Filling in your exercise plan for the following week, remembering to increase the numbers.
- Repeating your affirmations and affirmation questions.
- Doing a weekly planner for the week ahead. Remember to review your weekly planner to identify any patterns. Rejoice any achievements.
- Using the thoughts challenger sheet, particularly if you encounter any hurdles.
- Building up your enjoyable activities.
- Working towards your goals. Once you have achieved them, come up with new ones to further challenge you to greater achievement. Update your tracking sheet with what you learnt this week.

WEEK 7

A BETTER NIGHT'S SLEEP

How much sleep do we need for a good night's sleep? This varies from person to person. Some people need five hours a night, while others need eight to ten hours. The one thing that is common to most people with chronic pain is that they have difficulty sleeping.

Sometimes it is the pain that keeps you awake. Sometimes it is the fact that you may live a sedentary life and haven't used enough energy to feel tired. Sometimes pain medication has a side-effect of disturbing sleep patterns. And sometimes, your mind is too active for sleep to come easily.

Getting a good night's sleep replenishes your energy levels, enhances your mood and concentration levels, and most importantly, helps to manage your pain. If you find that you are not getting as much sleep as you need, below are some simple strategies that might help.

SEVEN WAYS TO A BETTER NIGHT'S SLEEP

Keep a sleep record
Each day in your logbook, make a list of the following:
- How long you were in bed.
- The number of times you woke up during the night.
- A number on a scale from 0 to10 to indicate how rested you felt in the morning (0 = no rest and 10 = well rested).
- Reasons why you might have had a good night's sleep or not.

Most people who keep a sleep record very quickly identify patterns. On days when they pace themselves with a healthy amount of activity and rest, they sleep better. On days when they don't pace themselves, or don't complete a relaxation technique, they might not sleep as well.

Have a regular routine before you go to bed

Try to go to sleep around the same time each night. It may be that you brush your teeth, turn the lights off, and perhaps do a relaxation session before you sleep. Avoid tea, coffee or other stimulants before bed, instead, try some warm milk or water. Avoid any activities that are mentally stimulating in bed such as watching TV or doing crossword puzzles.

Make the bedroom associated with sleeping

The aim here is to train your mind to recognise that your bedroom is a place of tranquillity and sleep. Avoid using your bedroom during the day, except when you are relaxing. Go to bed when you are sleepy and turn the lights off soon after. Create a peaceful and calming ambience in your bedroom; relaxing music, calming talks or incense will help.

The important thing is to associate your bedroom with sleeping. If you find you can't sleep, leave your bedroom for a while until you feel tired. You might listen to some calming music, read a book or try a visualisation technique.

Try to avoid paying attention to your clock

Move any clocks away from the bedroom. This will stop you from gazing at the clock or listening to the second hand ticking.

Challenge any unhelpful thoughts that come to your mind while in bed

If you are worried or stressed, or wake up in the middle of the night with thoughts in your mind, use a Thoughts

Challenger sheet and try to identify strategies to help you. Practice some of the relaxation techniques to help ease tension.

Establish a regular routine in the mornings and through the day
Wake up around the same time each morning. Some days will be more difficult, but ensure you stick to a routine. Avoid sleeping in, daytime naps or too much rest during the day. This will only make you lethargic and, at night, your sleep will be affected because you will have reserves of energy.

Consult your doctor
There are plenty of medications to help us sleep; some are prescribed by the doctor and some are natural and can be purchased over the counter. These can be helpful, but they are a short-term solution. Consult your doctor regarding what is best for you.

Weekly review
- If you have difficulty sleeping, complete a sleep record for a week in your logbook.
- Try some of the strategies listed above to help you sleep better.

And continue...
- Building on your daily activities.
- Being aware of your body and focusing on the gains.
- Pacing to an amount or time, not pain.
- Doing daily warm-ups and stretches.
- Exercising three times a week.
- Filling in your exercise plan for the following week, remembering to increase the numbers.

- Repeating your affirmations and affirmation questions.
- Doing a weekly planner for the week ahead. Remember to review your weekly planner to identify any patterns. Rejoice any achievements.
- Using the Thoughts Challenger sheet if you encounter any hurdles.
- Building up your enjoyable activities.
- Working towards your goals. Once you have achieved them, come up with new ones to further challenge you to greater achievement. Update your tracking sheet with what you learnt this week.
- Using relaxation techniques regularly.

WEEK 8

MANAGING FLARE-UPS AND SETBACKS

There will be times when your pain increases beyond normal levels. This is the nature of chronic pain. It is important to recognise this and have a plan to manage it as it happens. As discussed in Part 2 of this book, a flare-up is higher than normal pain levels that last for less than a couple of days. A setback is higher than normal pain levels that last for more than a couple of days.

A flare-up plan
The most common response to a flare-up is to immediately stop all activity. You may think that your stretches and exercises are causing the pain and stop doing them. But this is the worst thing you can do. As we have discussed a number of times, the body needs movement and activity to stay healthy and distract the mind from the pain. Rest is not the answer.

Regardless of the reason for the flare-up, the most important thing is to stick to your normal routine of stretches, exercises, relaxation, pacing and daily activities. Flare-ups will settle within a couple of days and it is important that your brain recognises that your body can function *normally* despite the flare-up. Try to avoid increasing your medication intake.

Once the flare-up has passed – which it will – reflect on possible triggers, the strategies that worked well in managing it, your thoughts and feelings during the experience, and what you can do to manage it better next time.

Analysing the flare-up can help you understand how your body responds. This is where your logbook is vital.

Read back over your activity levels in the days before the flare-up. While there might be no reason for the flare-up, there might be identifiable signs. Were you feeling angry and frustrated? Have you been more tired or stiffer in your muscles? Have you been sleeping properly? Have you suffered a stressful period in your life?

A setback plan
When a flare-up does not settle after a couple of days, this is a setback. During a setback it is not helpful to try to stick to your normal routine because all you will be doing is aggravating your pain and discomfort.

During a setback, assess what is happening and make notes in your logbook.

Cut all your activity levels by half for one week.

Once that week is over, use the next two weeks to build your activity back up to the level you were at before the setback. This will allow your body to rest and recharge to help manage the setback. This means cutting down your stretches and exercises, as well as your everyday activities.

At the end of the three-week adjustment period, look back over your logbook to see if there are any identifiable patterns to the setback. Also write down strategies that worked in managing the setback.

The important thing to note is that if you use a setback plan too often, its effectiveness reduces because your body becomes too used to it. It is important to keep it as the ace up your sleeve and only use it when things are really tough.

OVERCOMING PROBLEMS

When you begin some of your activities, you might come across some problems. You might not know where to begin your activities or may anticipate a flare-up. You might be convinced that something completely unexpected will happen.

You can ease your mind by planning ahead. A plan gives you confidence because it has strategies that help you through any situation. We call this a *Problem-solving plan*.

The following Problem-solving plan can be found at the back of this book, by scanning the QR code, or by visiting www.beyondpain.com.au and navigating to the 'Downloads' page.

Remember, it is not about trying to avoid a flare-up or setback. It is about having a plan and the confidence that, if you do have one, you will deal with it; you have had them before and you may have them in the future, but you will deal with them and take control.

Problem-solving plan

- Step 1: What is the problem?
    - Be as precise as possible:

    left knee pain while shopping

- Step 2: How is the problem affecting you?
    - How does it affect your thoughts and emotions?
    - What are your physical symptoms?
    - How does it affect your behaviour

    very frustrated
    knee feels hot, my frustration causes tension in my body
    I just lie down and rest when I have knee pain

- Step 3: Potential Strategies
    - Brainstorm a list of potential strategies from those taught in this book.

    Get someone to help with shopping
    Do shopping in two trips
    Take a couple of breaks during shopping
    Take some medication before I go
    Use a heat pack before and after my shopping
    Get a relaxation massage at the shopping centre

> *Cancel other plans that might make me tired on that day*

- Step 4: Plan

  - Pick the most appropriate and effective solutions and develop a plan of action. Include what strategies you need, and how, when, and where you would use them.

  Use a heat pack before and after

  Take 3 breaks (two coffee breaks, light lunch)– so that I pace myself

  Cancel other plans that might make me tired on that day

Weekly review

- Review your logbook and try and identify pain triggers and helpful practices.
- Fill out a Problem-solving plan for a situation that you are likely to encounter, or for a situation that was difficult to manage in the past. It may have been a flare-up or setback.

And continue...

- Building on your daily activities.
- Being aware of your body and focusing on the gains.
- Pacing to an amount or time, not pain.
- Doing daily warm-ups and stretches.
- Exercising three times a week.
- Filling in your exercise plan for the following week, remembering to increase the numbers.
- Repeating your affirmations and affirmation questions.
- Doing a weekly planner for the week ahead. Remember to review your weekly planner to identify any patterns. Rejoice any achievements.
- Using the Thoughts Challenger sheet if you encounter any hurdles.

- Building up your enjoyable activities.
- Working towards your goals. Once you have achieved them, come up with new ones to further challenge you to greater achievement. Update your tracking sheet with what you have learnt this week.
- Using relaxation techniques regularly.
- Reviewing your sleeping patterns and adopting helpful strategies.

THE FOUNDATION FOR A BETTER LIFE

As I stated earlier, the purpose of this program is to give you a choice – a choice to do what you want, when you want. A choice to say: *I could try that*, as opposed to: *no I can't do that.*

Choice is empowering.

Once you have completed this eight-week program, you will feel better, and have many choices available to you.

Once these strategies become habit, you can begin to rely less on writing everything down because you will have a better awareness of what works for you and what triggers your pain.

But don't become complacent at the end of the program. Keep your stretching routine going; this will keep your muscles and joints healthy. Build up your activity levels until you are enjoying life to the full. Make sure that you include things you want to do along with the things you have to do. As you become more active, you will not need to do the exercise program because you will be exercising during the course of your day.

Continue to use relaxation techniques because these help reduce pain and muscle spasms.

Continue to challenge any unhelpful thoughts. There may be times when you have thoughts that make you angry or upset, and that is normal. If these thoughts persist, challenge them until helpful thoughts become a habit.

Re-visit any of the exercises if you find yourself slipping back into unhelpful patterns. Remember that exercises are a great platform to get back to doing the things you really enjoy.

It will also be useful to read over the other strategies to remind yourself of what they are and how they can help. Teach someone else some of these strategies, because by teaching others, you will learn and refine the skills for yourself. Don't fall into the trap of just going over the strategies once and then not revising them.

Remember it is about staying focused and achieving your goals.

When you achieve your goals, find new ones to strive for using the strategies from this book.

I have used these strategies for over eight years and I no longer need to keep a logbook or complete an exercise program. I keep fit by swimming, hill climbing, kayaking and jogging – activities I enjoy. I still pace my activities, do my stretches and relaxation techniques. I don't even need to do regular Thought Challenger sheets, because I am now able to challenge unhelpful thinking in my head.

My flare-ups are fewer and my setbacks are rare.

Sometimes, I become complacent and think: *I can't be bothered, I'm doing okay so I don't need the strategies now.* Sometimes I get away with it, other times I don't. Sometimes, I overdo things and pay for it the next day. When I get like that, I remind myself to go back to basics: maintaining activity levels, using better pacing, doing more relaxation techniques and continuing my enjoyable activities.

These strategies have helped me to love, laugh, work and help others manage their pain, despite my own pain. They have allowed me to enjoy life, set goals, achieve them and set new more challenging ones.

My clients report the same. They no longer fear their pain, their flare-ups or their setbacks. They are confident that, no matter what happens, they have the strategies to manage. They achieve more of their goals and set more challenging ones. Pain is no longer their life, but just a small part of it.

Do this program and you too can live a life with purpose: a life beyond pain.

WORKSHEETS

Further copies can be downloaded for free by scanning the QR code, or by visiting www.beyondpain.com.au and navigating to the 'Downloads' page.

WEEK 1 – Weekly Planner

Weekly Planner (Please include approximate time you will do activity ; eg. shopping 1pm-2pm)	Monday	Tuesday	Wednesday	Thursday	Friday	Saturday	Sunday
Morning (5am – 12pm)							
Afternoon (12pm-5pm)							
Evening (5pm-10pm)							

WEEK 2 – GOAL SETTING: The 10-step goal sheet

Step	Steps to achieving the goal	Confidence rating (0–100%)
1	Increase your sitting tolerance in a car to 30 minutes	
2	Increase your sitting tolerance in a car to 1 hour of driving	
3	Increase your sitting tolerance in a car to 2 hours of driving	
4	Speak with your employer regarding suitable work options	
5	Be a passenger in a truck for two half days per week	
6	Be a passenger three half days per week	
7	Be a passenger on a part-time basis, three full days per week	
8	Drive a truck two half days per week	
9	Drive a truck two full days	
10	Returning to work part-time, working three full days as a truck driver	

WEEK 3 – EXERCISING: Exercise program

	Week __ of exercise					Week __ of exercise					Week __ of exercise				
	Mon	Tues	Wed	Thurs	Fri	Mon	Tues	Wed	Thurs	Fri	Mon	Tues	Wed	Thurs	Fri
Arm Circles Max 2mins or 40 circles															
Side Leans (max 10)															
Lunge Squats (max 15)															
Sit to Stands Max 40															
Chin Ins Max 10															
Tummy Tucks Max 10															
Back Arches Max10															
Sit Ups Max 30															
Scissor Legs Max10															
Tuck Ins Max 20															
Stairs/ Steps Max 30 steps															
Shoulder Presses Max 20															
Jogging Max 10 Mins															
Optional own Exercise															

WEEK 4 – THE RIGHT MINDSET: Perspective scale

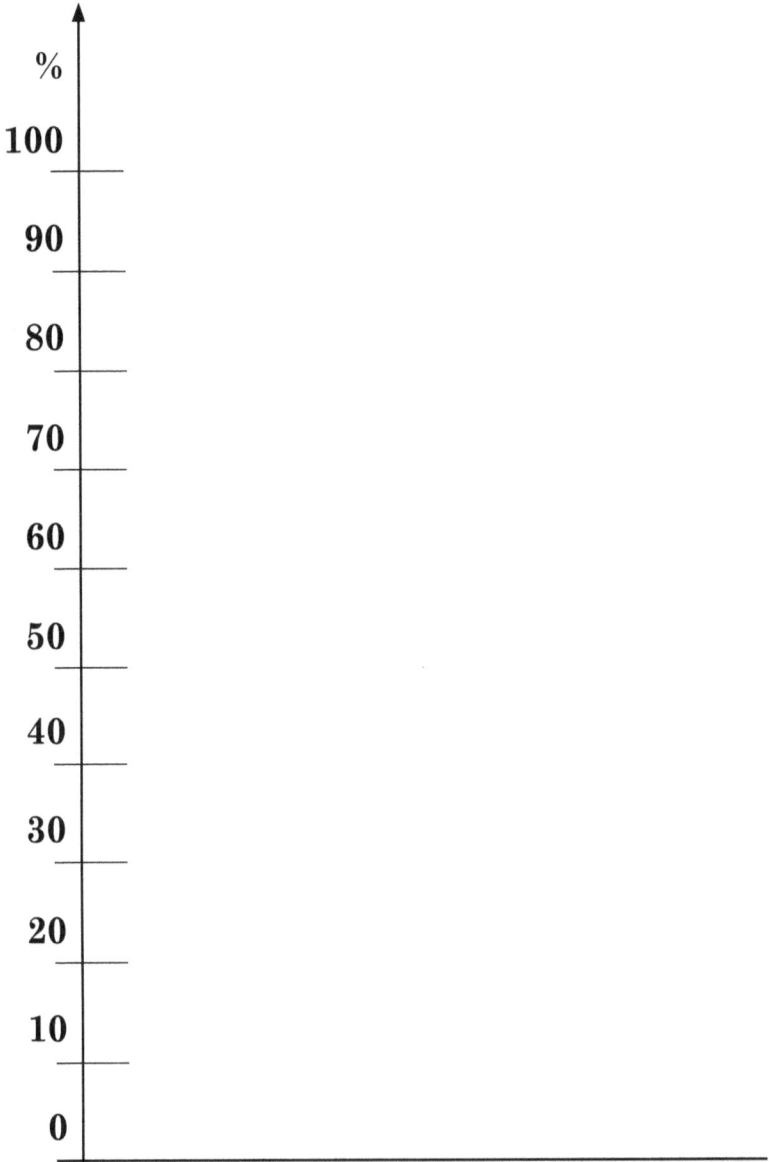

%

100

90

80

70

60

50

40

30

20

10

0

WEEK 4 – THE RIGHT MINDSET: Thoughts Challenger Sheet

Thoughts Challenger Sheet

- Think of a situation that has put you in a negative frame of mind.
- Fill in the three headings like the example.
- Ask yourself the four questions below.
- Fill in the three columns

Situation	Initial thoughts	Initial emotions

↓

Challenge your thoughts

The four questions

- Is it true?
- Is it helpful?
- Is it fair?
- What would you say to your best friend to encourage them if they were in your shoes?

Or ask an affirmation question:

- Why will I be able to finish vacuuming the whole house in the future?
- Why can I now do some of the vacuuming?

↓

More helpful thoughts	New emotions	Helpful behaviour and an action plan

WEEK 5 – KEEPING TRACK: Tracking Sheet

Week	Strategy	Goal 1	Goal 2
1	Affirmations Activity-relax cycle Journal		
2	Goal Setting Affirmation questions Stretch Program		
3	Exercises		
4	Challenging thoughts		
5	Enjoyable Activities		
6	Relaxation techniques		
7	Improving sleep		
8	Flare-up and setbacks: Problem-solving plan		

WEEK 8 – ADDRESSING PROBLEMS: Problem-solving plan

Problem-solving plan

- Step 1: What is the problem?
    - Be as precise as possible: *left knee pain while shopping*

    _____

    _____

    _____

- Step 2: How is the problem affecting you?
    - How does it affect your thoughts and emotions?
    - What are you physical symptoms?
    - How does it affect your behaviour

    _____

    _____

    _____

    _____

- Step 3: Potential Strategies
    - Brainstorm a list of potential strategies from those taught in this book.

    _____

    _____

    _____

    _____

- Step 4: Plan
    - Pick the most appropriate and effective solutions and develop a plan of action. Include the strategies you need, and how, when, and where you would use them.

    _____

    _____

    _____

REFERENCES

The following articles, used in this book, have been assessed by other researchers, experts in the field, and have been accepted as being scientifically valid. This means that you can trust the results and conclusions of these published studies.

Australasian Faculty of Occupational and Environmental Medicine 2011, *Australian and New Zealand consensus statement on the health benefits of work*, The Royal Australasian College of Physicians, October 2010.
My take: Health practitioner groups are now recognising the vast health benefits and supporting early return to work as an important part of the rehabilitation process.

Black, C 2008, 'Working for a healthier tomorrow: Dame Carol Black's review of the health of Britain's working age population', The Stationery Office, London.
My take: Working is good for us, physically, emotionally, economically and socially. We all need to take a fresh look at the health benefits of work and ensure we all do our part to promote a return to work.

Blyth, FM, March, LM, Nicholas, MK & Cousins, MJ 2003, 'Chronic pain, work performance and litigation', Pain, vol. 103, nos. 1–2, pp. 41–47.
My take: Most people with chronic pain are able to work and function normally and, therefore, complete relief from pain does not necessarily need to be the main goal of treatment. However, litigation (mainly work-related) for chronic pain is strongly associated with higher levels of pain-related disability, even after taking into account many other factors.

Boden, SD, Davis, DO, Dina, TS, Patronas, NJ & Wiesel, SW 1990, 'Abnormal magnetic-resonance scans of the lumbar spine in asymptomatic subjects. A prospective investigation', *Journal of Bone and Joint Surgery. American Volume*, vol. 72, no. 3, pp. 403–408.
My take: In this study of 67 subjects, it was normal to see bulging discs on the spines of people without pain. We must, therefore, interpret MRI findings taking into account age and clinical signs and symptoms. We shouldn't jump to conclusions based only on what an MRI scan shows.

Brox, JI, Nygaard, ØP, Holm, I & Keller, A, Ingebrigtsen, T & Reikerås, O 2010, 'Four-year follow-up of surgical versus non-surgical therapy for chronic low back pain', Annals of the Rheumatic Diseases, vol. 69, no. 9, pp. 1643–1648.
My take: Sometimes, further surgery is not the answer. In this study, people who had fusion surgery following failed disc surgery showed no more benefit than a more conservative approach using cognitive intervention and exercise.

Christoffersen, M 1994 'A follow-up study on the long term effects of unemployment on children: loss of self-esteem and self-destructive behaviour among adolescents', *Childhood*, vol. 2, no. 4, pp. 212–220.
My take: Unemployment of parents can have a significant negative effect on children when they grow up to become adults.

Coudeyre, E, Rannou, F, Tuback, F, Baron, G, Coriat, F, Brin, S, Revel, M & Poiraudeau, S 2006, 'General practitioners' fear-avoidance beliefs influence their management of patients with low back pain', *Pain*, vol. 124, no. 3, pp. 330–337.
My take: GP's own fears and assumptions about back pain can affect their ability to follow treatment guidelines, particularly those concerning occupational and physical activities.

Dunstan, DA 2009, 'Are sickness certificates doing our patients harm', *Australian Family Physician*, vol. 38, nos. 1–2, pp. 61–63.
My take: Issuing sickness certificates can have a negative effect on health and wellbeing. Treating practitioners need to have sound justification for issuing sickness certificates.

Edwards, RR, Almeida, DM, Klick, B, Haythornthwaite, JA & Smith, MT. 'Duration of sleep contributes to next-day pain report in the general population', *Pain*, vol. 137, no. 1, pp. 202–207.
My take: In this study, 971 participants were interviewed. Lack of sleep (or too much) can make your pain worse. If you have less than 6 hours (or more than 9 hours of sleep), your pain tends to be worse the next day.

Fullen, BM, Baxter, GD, O'Donovan, BG, Doody, C, Daly, L & Hurley, DA 2008, 'Doctors' attitudes and beliefs regarding acute low back pain management: a systematic review', *Pain*, vol. 136, no. 3, pp. 388–396.
My take: This paper reviewed research articles on the attitudes and beliefs of doctors. There was a lack of consensus regarding: the natural history of low back pain, treatment options and work-related issues. The lack of consensus and the attitudes and beliefs of General Practitioners need to change.

Indahl, A, Haldorsen, EH, Holm, S, Reikerås, O & Ursin, H 1998, 'Five-year follow-up study of a controlled clinical trial using light mobilization and an informative approach to low back pain', Spine (*Phila Pa 1976*), vol. 23, no. 23, pp. 2625–2630.
My take: In this study, 299 subjects were followed-up and the results suggest that sub-chronic low back pain can be managed successfully with a good clinical examination that is combined with education and provided in a manner designed to reduce fear and give reason to resume light activity.

Jensen, MC, Brant-Zawadzki, MN, Obuchowski, N, Modic, MT, Malkasian, D & Ross, JS 1994, 'Magnetic resonance imaging of the lumbar spine in people without back pain', *New England Journal of Medicine*, vol. 331, no. 2, pp. 69–73.
My take: Given the high prevalence of disc bulges and protrusions in people without back pain, MRI findings of bulges or protrusions in people with back pain could be coincidental.

Johnson, D & Fry, T 2002, 'Factors affecting return to work after injury: a study for the Victorian Work Cover Authority', *Melbourne Institute of Applied Economic and Social Research*, Melbourne.

My take: If you have 45 consecutive days off work (approximately 3 months), the likelihood of you ever returning to work drops to 50%. This can cause significant issues for the individual.

Leeuw, M, Goossens, ME, Linton, SJ, Crombez, G, Boersma, K & Vlaeyen, JW., 'The fear-avoidance model of musculoskeletal pain: current state of scientific evidence', *Journal of Behavioral Medicine*, vol. 30, no. 1, pp. 77–94.
My take: Fear avoidance behaviours can turn acute pain into a chronic pain condition without any further physical injury. We need to recognise how our emotional state can affect pain levels.

Lötters, FJ, Foets, M & Burdorf, A 2011, 'Work and health, a blind spot in curative healthcare? A pilot study', *Journal of Occupational Rehabilitation*, vol. 21, no. 3, pp. 304–312.
My take: In this study, visiting a medical specialist was seen to delay a return to work and resulted in higher pain intensity, lower functional ability and worse health perceptions. Visiting a physical therapist resulted in a faster return to work.

Malmivaara, A, Häkkinen, U, Aro, T, Heinrichs, ML, Koskenniemi, L, Kuosma, E, Lappi, S, Paloheimo, R, Servo, C, Vaaranen, V & Hernberg, S. 1995, 'The treatment of acute low back pain – bed rest, exercises, or ordinary activity?' *New England Journal of Medicine, vol. 332, no. 6, pp. 351–355.*
My take: Maintaining activity *within limits with relative rest breaks* leads to faster recovery than just bed rest or back-mobilising exercises

Marhold, C, Linton, SJ & Melin, L 2001, 'A cognitive-behavioral return-to-work program: effects on pain patients with a history of long-term versus short-term sick leave', *Pain*, vol. 91, nos. 1–2, pp. 155–163.
My take: If you want to get better sooner, you need to look at an early return-to-work focused rehabilitation program to prevent long-term sick leave or disability.

Moseley, GL 2004, 'Evidence for a direct relationship between cognitive and physical change during an education intervention in people with

chronic low back pain', *European Journal of Pain*, vol. 8, no. 1, pp. 39–45.
My take: In this study of 121 subjects, education sessions can change a person's unhelpful beliefs about pain and disability. By educating people, you can change their beliefs and behaviours, and help them become more confident in their own ability to become more active.

Moseley, GL, Nicholas, MK & Hodges, PW 2004, 'A randomized controlled trial of intensive neurophysiology education in chronic low back pain', *Clinical Journal of Pain*, vol. 20, no. 5, pp. 324–330.
My take: Education on pain neurophysiology, and not just about safe lifting, or how to keep your back strong and healthy, needs to be an integral part of treatment.

Moseley, L 2002, 'Combined physiotherapy and education is efficacious for chronic low back pain', *Australian Journal of Physiotherapy*, vol. 48, no. 4, pp. 297–302.
My take: This study of 57 subjects supports the use of combined physiotherapy and education for chronic low back pain.

Moseley, L 2003, 'Unravelling the barriers to reconceptualization of the problem in chronic pain: the actual and perceived ability of patients and health professionals to understand neurophysiology', *Journal of Pain*, vol. 4, no. 4, pp. 184–189.
My take: In this study of 276 patients and 288 professionals, both health professionals and patients could understand neurophysiology of pain but professionals underestimated the patients' ability to understand. The implications are that the poor knowledge of currently accurate information about pain and the underestimation of patients' ability to understand current accurate information about pain can represent barriers to effective rehabilitation.

Reinhardt Pedersen, C & Madsen M 2002, 'Parents' labour market participation as a predictor of children's health and wellbeing: a comparative study in five Nordic countries', *Journal of Epidemiology and Community Health*, vol. 56, no. 11, pp. 861–867.
My take: If you're not working for a long time, you can affect your children's perception of what is normal. This can result in them having a

high prevalence of ill health and low wellbeing.

Solantaus, T, Leinonen, J & Punamaki RL 2004, 'Children's mental health in times of economic recession: replication and extension of the family economic stress model in Finland', *Developmental Psychology*, vol. 40, no. 3, pp. 412–429.
My take: Economic stress and compromised parenting can result in children internalising and externalising stress-related symptoms. Having a balanced lifestyle is important.

Stadnik, TW, Lee, RR, Coen, HL, Neirynck, EC, Buisseret, TS & Osteaux, MJ 1998, 'Annular tears and disk herniation: prevalence and contrast enhancement on MR images in the absence of low back pain or sciatica', *Radiology*, vol. 206, no. 1, pp. 49–55.
My take: In this study of 36 asymptomatic subjects without low back pain or sciatica, annular tears and focal disc protrusions on MRI scans were frequently found.

Suter, PB 2002, 'Employment and litigation: improved by work, assisted by verdict', *Pain*, vol. 100, no. 3, pp. 249–257.
My take: This study recruited 200 subjects. Workers who return to work report less pain, less depression and less disability. Workers who are involved with litigation report more pain, greater depression and greater disability. Litigation seems to worsen the recovery, while early return to employment seems to improve recovery.

Tang, NK, Goodchild, CE, Hester, J & Salkovskis, PM 2010, 'Mental defeat is linked to interference, distress and disability in chronic pain', *Pain*, vol. 149, no. 3, pp. 547–554.
My take: In the 133 subjects who participated in the study, mental defeat was strongly related to pain levels, sleep disturbances, anxiety, depression, functional and psychosocial disability.

Vlaeyen JW & Linton SJ 2000, 'Fear-avoidance and its consequences in chronic musculoskeletal pain: a state of the art', *Pain*, vol. 85, no. 3, pp. 317–332.
My take: Pain-related fear and avoidance might be a crucial feature of

the development of a chronic problem for people with musculoskeletal pain.

Waddell, G & Burton, AK 2006, *Is work good for your health and well-being?* The Stationery Office, London.
My take: The health benefits of work seem to outweigh work absenteeism. Being off work for long periods appears to have a negative effect on health.

Wiesel, SW, Tsourmas, N, Feffer, HL, Citrin, CM & Patronas, N 1984, 'A study of computer-assisted tomography. I. The incidence of positive CAT scans in an asymptomatic group of patients', *Spine (Phila Pa 1976)*, vol. 9, no. 6, pp. 549–551.
My take: In this study, 52 scans from a control group with no history of back trouble were mixed with 6 scans of patients proven to have spinal disease. The results indicate that even in asymptomatic subjects, there can be significant radiological findings.

NOTES:

www.ingramcontent.com/pod-product-compliance
Lightning Source LLC
Chambersburg PA
CBHW030633270326

41929CB00007B/65